AF798426

Instruction *Donum Vitae*

Preface
Cardinal Joseph Ratzinger Later Pope Ben-16

Instruction on Respect for Human Life in Its Origin and on the Dignity of Procreation

Commentaries and Studies
M. Schooyans—A.R. Luño—B. Kiely—A. Scola
D. Tettamanzi—A. Chapelle—E. Sgreccia—G. Mémeteau

On the Doctrinal Authority of the Instruction "Donum Vitae"

Libreria Editrice Vaticana
United States Conference of Catholic Bishops
Washington, DC

English translation copyright © 2013, Libreria Editrice Vaticana (LEV). All rights reserved. Article by Kiely, copyright © 1987, LEV. Used with permission.

Quotations from *Code of Canon Law: Latin-English Edition: New English Translation* (*Codex Iuris Canonici* [CIC]) copyright © 1998, Canon Law Society of America, Washington, DC. Used with permission. All rights reserved.

Scripture excerpts used in this work are taken from the *New American Bible*, rev. ed. © 2010, 1991, 1986, 1970 Confraternity of Christian Doctrine, Inc., Washington, DC. All rights reserved.

Excerpts from *The Documents of Vatican II*, Walter M. Abbott, SJ, General Editor, copyright © 1966 by America Press, Inc. Reprinted with permission. All rights reserved.

English translation of *Istruzione <<Donum Vitae>> Su il rispetto della vita umana nascente el la dignità della procreazione* [Documenti e Studi 12], LEV, 1990.

Cover image, iStockphoto.

ISBN 978-1-60137-296-3

First printing, August 2013

Contents

Preface

The Instruction *Donum Vitae: On Respect for Human Life in Its Origin and on the Dignity of Procreation*, published February 22, 1987, has witnessed a large reaction among pastors, the faithful, and—thanks to mass media—in a large part public and even non-Catholic opinion. There have been many and qualified expressions of agreement, although there have also been those of misunderstanding and opposition. The Congregation for the Doctrine of the Faith has considered it helpful to publish, in a bound volume such as is used for its principle documents, the text of the Instruction itself, along with a series of commentaries that appeared at the same time in *L'Osservatore Romano*. The hope is thus to encourage the spread of these studies with the goal of facilitating a serene and profound reflection regarding such an important theme of the Church's moral doctrine.

Before moving on to the presentation of the contents, I think it necessary to say a word on the literary genre of the present Instruction: it does not attempt to elaborate an organic or complete treatment on the Church's teaching concerning the dignity of nascent human life and procreation. Nor does the document pretend to offer a complete depiction of all the concrete case studies that surface in this area. The goal of the Instruction is much more modest: it attempts—as the subtitle says—to simply present the responses of Catholic moral doctrine to certain particularly relevant questions regarding new possibilities of intervention, which man has acquired through biomedical technology, in the initial phases of the life of the human being, and in the very processes of procreation.

The Congregation for the Doctrine of the Faith has received related questions from different episcopal conferences and individual bishops, from theologians and doctors, from men of science, and from married couples. The present Instruction, which is the fruit of an enormous amount of consultation and of long and meditative research, therefore offers specific answers to the main contemporary questions on this matter. Nevertheless, these answers are not merely a neat exposition from within a coherent logical framework but fundamentally depend on an anthropology—that is, a vision of man, of his nature and his dignity, of his origins and his destiny—that serves as the basis for the different ethical cases that are dealt with here. Outside this vision of man the individual responses to the multifaceted case studies will be incomprehensible.

For this reason, before entering into the details of the contents, I want to direct attention to an essential aspect that can easily become obscured, that is, to the vision of the human person, which is summarily portrayed, above all in the Introduction.

It must also be noted that the anthropology of the present Instruction, although briefly presented, reiterates the Church's prior teaching with profound continuity and harmony.

1) The first thesis of this vision of man consists in the affirmation of the substantial unity of the human person. This is a very important thesis, both in itself and in relation to the present cultural context.

The human body is a constitutive part of the person, through which he manifests and expresses himself. Thanks to the union with the spirit, the body is the manifestation of the person himself. One could also say that the body is the person himself in his visibility. This yields decisive consequences both on the anthropological and the ethical level. As to the anthropological level, although from a purely scientific perspective the human body can be viewed and treated as a complex of tissues, organs, and functions, along the same lines as the bodies of animals, to someone looking with metaphysical and theological eyes things appear essentially otherwise: the human body is indeed situated on a qualitatively superior plane of being. As to the ethical level, the respect owed to the person must be expressed as a respect also for the human body, through which the person expresses himself.

The Church's recalling of this central truth has become particularly important today. Despite appearances, there is a profound devaluation of the body, which is considered as simply an "object" of which one can make use. This reductive conception of the body is inevitably accompanied by a devaluation of the person.

2) The second thesis, which lies at the base of the preceding one and to which the Church can never direct enough attention, is the following: the human person is endowed with such dignity that he can never be considered or treated as an "object" but always and only as a "subject." He is not "something" but "someone." This thesis has already been placed at the center of the recent Instructions *On Certain Aspects of Liberation Theology* and *On Christian Freedom and Liberation*; the present Instruction is situated in ideal continuity with these recent documents from the Congregation for the Doctrine of the Faith. The intrinsic logic of many contemporary reproductive techniques is a logic of "the production of objects," a logic that inherently establishes a relationship of inequality between the technician (who produces) and that

which is produced, and therefore a relationship of domination by one over the other.

Here we find a particular application of the "preferential love for the poor," which the second Instruction of the Congregation for the Doctrine of the Faith, *On Christian Freedom and Liberation* (no. 68), has recognized as an essential aspect of the Church's evangelical witness. Indeed, who is more poor and defenseless, more in need of protection, more exposed to the abuses of those with power, than the human being newly formed and not yet born?

The word of Christ, which appears in the last phrase of our document, finds here a new and particular resonance, "What you do to one of the least of my brethren, you do unto me" (Mt 25:40).

In order to understand the unacceptability of this logic of production as applied to human procreation, we must free ourselves from one of the most lamentable beliefs that this "technology" has itself introduced into our consciousness: the idea that reality does not possess a truth of its own, but that the *intention* of man, and that alone, creates an ontological meaning for everything. Indeed, the difficulty that continually counteracts the Church's teaching (and that will certainly counteract the present Instruction as well) is drawn from the subjective *intentions* (desires) of those involved in these processes (spouses, doctors); the intention (desire) of the spouses to have a child and the intention of the researchers and doctors to increase their own knowledge for the future benefit of humanity are basically good, morally laudable intentions. The Church deeply grasps the legitimate aspirations of the spouses to see the sign of their conjugal love expressed in a child. The Church appreciates, moreover, the impetus for medical research to cure conjugal sterility; it already encourages such development and celebrates the positive results already attained, as long as the dignity of human procreation is fully safeguarded. Nonetheless, the uprightness of the end and the goodness of the subjective intentions do not alone suffice to render licit, from the moral point of view, the recourse to whatever means biomedical technology today places at our disposal. What is technically possible is not in itself also morally admissible. This is why the Church's Magisterium cannot descend to even the smallest compromise with a vision in which subjective desire is the sole and sufficient criterion for legitimizing any medical intervention. Such a conception is ultimately rooted in the denial of the truth of creation. Furthermore, one may point out that even certain widespread diagnoses regarding the contemporary cultural situation—although they begin from quite different presuppositions—agree with the Catholic Church in this judgment about the essentially anti-human character of the productive-technological mentality.

This second anthropological thesis confronts a central question in all the subject matter addressed by the Instruction: what is the act which by its nature is ethically worthy to establish the conditions for conceiving a new human person? The document's third anthropological-ethical thesis replies to this question.

3) The third thesis is consequently the following: only the conjugal act is worthy to establish the conditions for conceiving a new human person.

To understand the basis of this thesis, it is, in the first place, necessary to integrate it within the general Christian vision of human sexuality. This vision has found recent expression in the Pastoral Constitution *Gaudium et Spes*, in the Encyclical *Humanae Vitae*, in the Apostolic Exhortation *Familiaris Consortio*, and the catecheses of the Holy Father on human love. A unique anthropological conception of sexuality, ever deepening, links these documents to each other and to the present Instruction. It is well to briefly review it.

Conjugal sexuality is the expression of the definitive gift that the spouse makes *of himself* to the other, and as such confirms and aids in the spouses a communion of total and indissoluble love. It is because of this, its intimate truth, that conjugal sexuality, precisely in the specific conjugal act of the spouses' union, is called to a *participationem specialem quamdam in suiipsius opera creativo* (namely, God's) (*Gaudium et Spes*, no. 50, par. 1). It is therefore neither *by chance* nor as a pure *fact of life* that these two fundamental meanings—the unitive and the procreative—reside in the conjugal act. This "cohabitation," or connection, is a *moral requirement* based on the very nature of man and on his relationship with God the Creator. It is an onto-axiological requirement. Consequently, this connection between the unitive meaning and the procreative meaning of the conjugal act may never be broken, as *Humanae Vitae* (no. 12) teaches.

The conjugal act, in which are established the conditions for the emergence of a new life, does not institute a "production" relationship between parents and children; children are generated in it, not produced. The spouses situate an act of love within the reciprocal gift of themselves, and the child who may emerge from this act is the gift of God's creative love, entrusted to the parents that they might welcome him with recognition and with infinite respect.

We can see then that there is an intrinsic coherence between all these truths, and that this vision of man possesses an admirable internal harmony.

Every person deserves unconditional respect, and can never be reduced to an object of use: this principle applies from conception until death. For this reason the conjugal act, in which the spouses express their communion of interpersonal love in a specific way, is the sole "cradle" worthy of the new human being.

An authentic and profound understanding of these three foundational theses will enable the derivation of criteria for the solution of the various cases addressed in the document.

Final Observations

It does not seem amiss to conclude with some more particular reflections for the sake of a better understanding of the document.

1) The Instruction, more than any other preceding magisterial document, enters an "area of overlap" between anthropology, ethics, science, and technology. From this perspective the document might be sophistically attacked or misunderstood for two reasons: science's claim to autonomy, and the many places where the document says "no."

Regarding the first objection, some reflections are in order. The battle for science's autonomy is today a "rearguard action," so to speak. Indeed, if by the autonomy of science one means to state that it is endowed with its own proper epistemology (with its own object of study and its own methods of research), then we are speaking of something that is today so taken for granted that only a "prejudice" could bring the discussion to this point. If, however, "autonomy" is in fact used to reduce the humanity of the scientist to his role as scientist, then we must make a clarification. Scientific activity, insofar as it is human activity, is subject to ethical laws; science is not some absolute to which everything, even human dignity, should be subordinated and eventually sacrificed. Today all men—believers and non-believers—who consider the destinies of humanity are worried by this "reduction" and by this subordination of human values to scientific logic. One need only think of the ecological problem, or the problem of nuclear energy. The real issue, today more than ever, is how to integrate science within an authentically human culture. In this sense there is talk of a "rearguard attitude" with respect to those persons who worry only about autonomy. And thus it should be understood that the "nos" directed toward certain experiments and certain reproductive techniques are really a "yes" said to man, a witness to man's dignity and salvation.

2) In the light of the previous considerations, it should be understood how the Instruction indicates an urgent and necessary task for theologians and moralists in particular.

In order to render the contents of the magisterial teaching more profound and ever more accessible to the faithful, it is necessary to elaborate a valid anthropology in matters of sexuality and matrimony, and through a properly interdisciplinary approach. In the context of a facilely pragmatic and utilitarian culture, which evaluates the morality of human actions only on the basis of their results, there is the indispensable need for an ethical reflection capable of showing the irreducible originality of the moral good and its rootedness in the entire truth about man that reason, illuminated by faith, discovers. It is the task of moral theology to show that the existence of moral norms, with a precise, immutable, and unconditional content, is the only guarantee for the respect and the full realization of man in his truth.

Given this task of more fundamental anthropological and ethical reflection, in fidelity to the Church's Magisterium and in renewed creativity, moral theology will increasingly discover its identity and its own worth: that of contributing toward, that is, securing for the humanity of tomorrow, the possibility of living and loving in that dignity and freedom which comes from the respect for the truth, and of working for the defense and promotion of man, for his eternal salvation, and therefore, ultimately for the glory of God.

Joseph Cardinal Ratzinger

Instruction on Respect for Human Life in Its Origin and on the Dignity of Procreation

Replies to Certain Questions of the Day

Foreword

The Congregation for the Doctrine of the Faith has been approached by various Episcopal Conferences or individual Bishops, by theologians, doctors and scientists, concerning biomedical techniques which make it possible to intervene in the initial phase of the life of a human being and in the very processes of procreation and their conformity with the principles of Catholic morality. The present Instruction, which is the result of wide consultation and in particular of a careful evaluation of the declarations made by Episcopates, does not intend to repeat all the Church's teaching on the dignity of human life as it originates and on procreation, but to offer, in the light of the previous teaching of the Magisterium, some specific replies to the main questions being asked in this regard. The exposition is arranged as follows: an introduction will recall the fundamental principles, of an anthropological and moral character, which are necessary for a proper evaluation of the problems and for working out replies to those questions; the first part will have as its subject respect for the human being from the first moment of his or her existence; the second part will deal with the moral questions raised by technical interventions on human procreation; the third part will offer some orientations on the relationships between moral law and civil law in terms of the respect due to human embryos and fetuses* and as regards the legitimacy of techniques of artificial procreation.

* The terms "zygote," "pre-embryo," "embryo," and "fetus" can indicate in the vocabulary of biology successive stages of the development of a human being. The present Instruction makes free use of these terms, attributing to them an identical ethical relevance, in order to designate the result (whether visible or not) of human generation, from the first moment of its existence until birth. The reason for this usage is clarified by the text (cf. I, 1).

Introduction

1. Biomedical Research and the Teaching of the Church

The gift of life which God the Creator and Father has entrusted to man calls him to appreciate the inestimable value of what he has been given and to take responsibility for it: this fundamental principle must be placed at the center of one's reflection in order to clarify and solve the moral problems raised by artificial interventions on life as it originates and on the processes of procreation.

Thanks to the progress of the biological and medical sciences, man has at his disposal ever more effective therapeutic resources; but he can also acquire new powers, with unforeseeable consequences, over human life at its very beginning and in its first stages. Various procedures now make it possible to intervene not only in order to assist but also to dominate the processes of procreation. These techniques can enable man to "take in hand his own destiny," but they also expose him "to the temptation to go beyond the limits of a reasonable dominion over nature."[1] They might constitute progress in the service of man, but they also involve serious risks. Many people are therefore expressing an urgent appeal that in interventions on procreation the values and rights of the human person be safeguarded. Requests for clarification and guidance are coming not only from the faithful but also from those who recognize the Church as "an expert in humanity"[2] with a mission to serve the "civilization of love"[3] and of life.

The Church's Magisterium does not intervene on the basis of a particular competence in the area of the experimental sciences; but having taken account of the data of research and technology, it intends to put forward, by virtue of its evangelical mission and apostolic duty, the moral teaching corresponding to the dignity of the person and to his or her integral vocation. It intends to do so by expounding the criteria of moral judgment as regards the applications of scientific research and technology, especially in relation to human life and its beginnings. These criteria are the respect, defense and promotion of man, his "primary and fundamental right" to life,[4] his dignity as

1 Pope John Paul II, *Discourse to those taking part in the 81st Congress of the Italian Society of Internal Medicine and the 82nd Congress of the Italian Society of General Surgery*, October 27, 1980: AAS 72 (1980) 1126.

2 Pope Paul VI, *Discourse to the General Assembly of the United Nations Organization*, October 4, 1965: AAS 57 (1965) 878; Encyclical *Populorum Progressio*, no. 13: AAS 59 (1967) 263.

3 Pope Paul VI, *Homily during the Mass closing the Holy Year*, December 25, 1975: AAS 68 (1976) 145; Pope John Paul II, Encyclical *Dives in Misericordia*, no. 30: AAS 72 (1980) 1224.

4 Pope John Paul II, *Discourse to those taking part in the 35th General Assembly of the World*

a person who is endowed with a spiritual soul and with moral responsibility[5] and who is called to beatific communion with God.

The Church's intervention in this field is inspired also by the Love which she owes to man, helping him to recognize and respect his rights and duties. This love draws from the fount of Christ's love: as she contemplates the mystery of the Incarnate Word, the Church also comes to understand the "mystery of man";[6] by proclaiming the Gospel of salvation, she reveals to man his dignity and invites him to discover fully the truth of his own being. Thus the Church once more puts forward the divine law in order to accomplish the work of truth and liberation.

For it is out of goodness—in order to indicate the path of life—that God gives human beings his commandments and the grace to observe them: and it is likewise out of goodness—in order to help them persevere along the same path—that God always offers to everyone his forgiveness. Christ has compassion on our weaknesses: he is our Creator and Redeemer. May his spirit open men's hearts to the gift of God's peace and to an understanding of his precepts.

2. Science and Technology at the Service of the Human Person

God created man in his own image and likeness: "Male and female he created them" (Gn 1:27), entrusting to them the task of "having dominion over the earth" (Gn 1:28). Basic scientific research and applied research constitute a significant expression of this dominion of man over creation. Science and technology are valuable resources for man when placed at his service and when they promote his integral development for the benefit of all; but they cannot of themselves show the meaning of existence and of human progress. Being ordered to man, who initiates and develops them, they draw from the person and his moral values the indication of their purpose and the awareness of their limits.

It would on the one hand be illusory to claim that scientific research and its applications are morally neutral; on the other hand one cannot derive criteria for guidance from mere technical efficiency, from research's possible usefulness to some at the expense of others, or, worse still, from prevailing ideologies. Thus science and technology require, for their own intrinsic meaning, an unconditional respect for the fundamental criteria of the moral law: that

---

Medical Association, October 29, 1983: AAS 76 (1984) 390.

5 Cf. Declaration *Dignitatis Humanae*, no. 2.

6 Pastoral Constitution *Gaudium et Spes*, no. 22; Pope John Paul II, Encyclical *Redemptor Hominis*, no. 8: AAS 71 (1979) 270-272.

is to say, they must be at the service of the human person, of his inalienable rights and his true and integral good according to the design and will of God.[7]

The rapid development of technological discoveries gives greater urgency to this need to respect the criteria just mentioned: science without conscience can only lead to man's ruin. "Our era needs such wisdom more than bygone ages if the discoveries made by man are to be further humanized. For the future of the world stands in peril unless wiser people are forthcoming."[8]

3. *Anthropology and Procedures in the Biomedical Field*

Which moral criteria must be applied in order to clarify the problems posed today in the field of biomedicine? The answer to this question presupposes a proper idea of the nature of the human person in his bodily dimension.

For it is only in keeping with his true nature that the human person can achieve self-realization as a "unified totality":[9] and this nature is at the same time corporal and spiritual. By virtue of its substantial union with a spiritual soul, the human body cannot be considered as a mere complex of tissues, organs and functions, nor can it be evaluated in the same way as the body of animals; rather it is a constitutive part of the person who manifests and expresses himself through it.

The natural moral law expresses and lays down the purposes, rights and duties which are based upon the bodily and spiritual nature of the human person. Therefore this law cannot be thought of as simply a set of norms on the biological level; rather it must be defined as the rational order whereby man is called by the Creator to direct and regulate his life and actions and in particular to make use of his own body.[10]

A first consequence can be deduced from these principles: an intervention on the human body affects not only the tissues, the organs and their functions but also involves the person himself on different levels. It involves, therefore, perhaps in an implicit but nonetheless real way, a moral significance and responsibility. Pope John Paul II forcefully reaffirmed this to the World Medical Association when he said: "Each human person, in his absolutely unique singularity, is constituted not only by his spirit, but by his body

7 Cf. Pastoral Constitution *Gaudium et Spes*, no. 35.

8 Pastoral Constitution *Gaudium et Spes*, no. 15; cf. also Pope Paul VI, Encyclical *Populorum Progressio*, no. 20: AAS 59 (1967) 267; Pope John Paul II, Encyclical *Redemptor Hominis*, no. 15: AAS 71 (1979) 286-289; Apostolic Exhortation *Familiaris Consortio*, no. 8: AAS 74 (1982) 89.

9 Pope John Paul II, Apostolic Exhortation *Familiaris Consortio*, no. 11: AAS 74 (1982) 92.

10 Cf. Pope Paul VI, Encyclical *Humanae Vitae*, no. 10: AAS 60 (1968) 487-488.

as well. Thus, in the body and through the body, one touches the person himself in his concrete reality. To respect the dignity of man consequently amounts to safeguarding this identity of the man *corpore et anima unus*, as the Second Vatican Council says (*Gaudium et Spes*, no. 14, par.1). It is on the basis of this anthropological vision that one is to find the fundamental criteria for decision-making in the case of procedures which are not strictly therapeutic, as, for example, those aimed at the improvement of the human biological condition."[11]

Applied biology and medicine work together for the integral good of human life when they come to the aid of a person stricken by illness and infirmity and when they respect his or her dignity as a creature of God. No biologist or doctor can reasonably claim, by virtue of his scientific competence, to be able to decide on people's origin and destiny. This norm must be applied in a particular way in the field of sexuality and procreation, in which man and woman actualize the fundamental values of love and life.

God, who is love and life, has inscribed in man and woman the vocation to share in a special way in his mystery of personal communion and in his work as Creator and Father.[12] For this reason marriage possesses specific goods and values in its union and in procreation which cannot be likened to those existing in lower forms of life. Such values and meanings are of the personal order and determine from the moral point of view the meaning and limits of artificial interventions on procreation and on the origin of human life. These interventions are not to be rejected on the grounds that they are artificial. As such, they bear witness to the possibilities of the art of medicine. But they must be given a moral evaluation in reference to the dignity of the human person, who is called to realize his vocation from God to the gift of love and the gift of life.

4. *Fundamental Criteria for a Moral Judgment*

The fundamental values connected with the techniques of artificial human procreation are two: the life of the human being called into existence and the special nature of the transmission of human life in marriage. The moral judgment on such methods of artificial procreation must therefore be formulated in reference to these values.

Physical life, with which the course of human life in the world begins, certainly does not itself contain the whole of a person's value, nor does it

---

11 Pope John Paul II, *Discourse to the members of the 35th General Assembly of the World Medical Association*, October 29, 1983: AAS 76 (1984) 393.

12 Cf. Pope John Paul II, Apostolic Exhortation *Familiaris Consortio*, no. 11: AAS 74 (1982) 91-92; cf. also Pastoral Constitution *Gaudium et Spes*, no. 50.

represent the supreme good of man who is called to eternal life. However it does constitute in a certain way the "fundamental" value of life, precisely because upon this physical life all the other values of the person are based and developed.[13] The inviolability of the innocent human being's right to life "from the moment of conception until death"[14] is a sign and requirement of the very inviolability of the person to whom the Creator has given the gift of life.

By comparison with the transmission of other forms of life in the universe, the transmission of human life has a special character of its own, which derives from the special nature of the human person. "The transmission of human life is entrusted by nature to a personal and conscious act and as such is subject to the all-holy laws of God: immutable and inviolable laws which must be recognized and observed. For this reason one cannot use means and follow methods which could be licit in the transmission of the life of plants and animals."[15]

Advances in technology have now made it possible to procreate apart from sexual relations through the meeting *in vitro* of the germ-cells previously taken from the man and the woman. But what is technically possible is not for that very reason morally admissible. Rational reflection on the fundamental values of life and of human procreation is therefore indispensable for formulating a moral evaluation of such technological interventions on a human being from the first stages of his development.

5. *Teachings of the Magisterium*

On its part, the Magisterium of the Church offers to human reason in this field too the light of Revelation: the doctrine concerning man taught by the Magisterium contains many elements which throw light on the problems being faced here.

From the moment of conception, the life of every human being is to be respected in an absolute way because man is the only creature on earth that God has "wished for himself"[16] and the spiritual soul of each man is "immediately created" by God;[17] his whole being bears the image of the Creator.

13 Sacred Congregation for the Doctrine of the Faith, *Declaration on Procured Abortion*, 9, AAS 66 (1974) 736-737.

14 Pope John Paul II, *Discourse to those taking part in the 35th General Assembly of the World Medical Association*, October 29, 1983: AAS 76 (1984) 390.

15 Pope John XXIII, Encyclical *Mater et Magistra*, III: AAS 53 (1961) 447.

16 Pastoral Constitution *Gaudium et Spes*, no. 24.

17 Cf. Pope Pius XII, Encyclical *Humani Generis*: AAS 42 (1950) 575; Pope Paul VI, *Professio*

Human life is sacred because from its beginning it involves "the creative action of God"[18] and it remains forever in a special relationship with the Creator, who is its sole end.[19] God alone is the Lord of life from its beginning until its end: no one can, in any circumstance, claim for himself the right to destroy directly an innocent human being.[20]

Human procreation requires on the part of the spouses responsible collaboration with the fruitful love of God;[21] the gift of human life must be actualized in marriage through the specific and exclusive acts of husband and wife, in accordance with the laws inscribed in their persons and in their union.[22]

I. Respect for Human Embryos

Careful reflection on this teaching of the Magisterium and on the evidence of reason, as mentioned above, enables us to respond to the numerous moral problems posed by technical interventions upon the human being in the first phases of his life and upon the processes of his conception.

1. What respect is due to the human embryo, taking into account his nature and identity?

The human being must be respected—as a person—from the very first instant of his existence.

The implementation of procedures of artificial fertilization has made possible various interventions upon embryos and human fetuses. The aims pursued are of various kinds: diagnostic and therapeutic, scientific and commercial.

Fidei: AAS 60 (1968) 436.

18 Pope John XXIII, Encyclical *Mater et Magistra*, III: AAS 53 (1961) 447; cf. Pope John Paul II, *Discourse to priests participating in a seminar on "Responsible Procreation,"* September 17, 1983, *Insegnamenti di Giovanni Paolo II*, VI, 2 (1983) 562: "At the origin of each human person there is a creative act of God: no man comes into existence by chance; he is always the result of the creative love of God."

19 Cf. Pastoral Constitution *Gaudium et Spes*, no. 24.

20 Cf. Pope Pius XII, *Discourse to the Saint Luke Medical-Biological Union*, November 12, 1944: *Discorsi e Radiomessaggi* VI (1944-1945) 191-192.

21 Cf. Pastoral Constitution *Gaudium et Spes*, no. 50.

22 Cf. Pastoral Constitution *Gaudium et Spes*, no. 51: "When it is a question of harmonizing married love with the responsible transmission of life, the moral character of one's behavior does not depend only on the good intention and the evaluation of the motives: the objective criteria must be used, criteria drawn from the nature of the human person and human acts, criteria which respect the total meaning of mutual self-giving and human procreation in the context of true love."

From all of this, serious problems arise. Can one speak of a right to experimentation upon human embryos for the purpose of scientific research? What norms or laws should be worked out with regard to this matter? The response to these problems presupposes a detailed reflection on the nature and specific identity—the word "status" is used—of the human embryo itself.

At the Second Vatican Council, the Church for her part presented once again to modern man her constant and certain doctrine according to which: "Life once conceived, must be protected with the utmost care; abortion and infanticide are abominable crimes."[23] More recently, the *Charter of the Rights of the Family*, published by the Holy See, confirmed that "human life must be absolutely respected and protected from the moment of conception."[24]

This Congregation is aware of the current debates concerning the beginning of human life, concerning the individuality of the human being and concerning the identity of the human person. The Congregation recalls the teachings found in the *Declaration on Procured Abortion*: "From the time that the ovum is fertilized, a new life is begun which is neither that of the father nor of the mother; it is rather the life of a new human being with his own growth. It would never be made human if it were not human already. To this perpetual evidence . . . modern genetic science brings valuable confirmation. It has demonstrated that, from the first instant, the program is fixed as to what this living being will be: a man, this individual-man with his characteristic aspects already well determined. Right from fertilization is begun the adventure of a human life, and each of its great capacities requires time . . . to find its place and to be in a position to act."[25] This teaching remains valid and is further confirmed, if confirmation were needed, by recent findings of human biological science which recognize that in the zygote[*] resulting from fertilization the biological identity of a new human individual is already constituted.

Certainly no experimental datum can be in itself sufficient to bring us to the recognition of a spiritual soul; nevertheless, the conclusions of science regarding the human embryo provide a valuable indication for discerning by the use of reason a personal presence at the moment of this first appearance of a human life: how could a human individual not be a human person? The Magisterium has not expressly committed itself to an affirmation of a philosophical nature, but it constantly reaffirms the moral condemnation

* The zygote is the cell produced when the nuclei of the two gametes have fused.

23 Pastoral Constitution *Gaudium et Spes*, no. 51.

24 Holy See, *Charter of the Rights of the Family*, 4: *L'Osservatore Romano*, November 25, 1983.

25 Sacred Congregation for the Doctrine of the Faith, *Declaration on Procured Abortion*, 12-13: AAS 66 (1974) 738.

of any kind of procured abortion. This teaching has not been changed and is unchangeable.[26]

Thus the fruit of human generation, from the first moment of its existence, that is to say from the moment the zygote has formed, demands the unconditional respect that is morally due to the human being in his bodily and spiritual totality. The human being is to be respected and treated as a person from the moment of conception; and therefore from that same moment his rights as a person must be recognized, among which in the first place is the inviolable right of every innocent human being to life.

This doctrinal reminder provides the fundamental criterion for the solution of the various problems posed by the development of the biomedical sciences in this field: since the embryo must be treated as a person, it must also be defended in its integrity, tended and cared for, to the extent possible, in the same way as any other human being as far as medical assistance is concerned.

2. Is prenatal diagnosis morally licit?

If prenatal diagnosis respects the life and integrity of the embryo and the human fetus and is directed toward its safeguarding or healing as an individual, then the answer is affirmative.

For prenatal diagnosis makes it possible to know the condition of the embryo and of the fetus when still in the mother's womb. It permits, or makes it possible to anticipate earlier and more effectively, certain therapeutic, medical or surgical procedures.

Such diagnosis is permissible, with the consent of the parents after they have been adequately informed, if the methods employed safeguard the life and integrity of the embryo and the mother, without subjecting them to disproportionate risks.[27] But this diagnosis is gravely opposed to the moral law

---

26 Cf. Pope Paul VI, *Discourse to participants in the Twenty-third National Congress of Italian Catholic Jurists*, December 9, 1972: AAS 64 (1972) 777.

27 The obligation to avoid disproportionate risks involves an authentic respect for human beings and the uprightness of therapeutic intentions. It implies that the doctor "above all . . . must carefully evaluate the possible negative consequences which the necessary use of a particular exploratory technique may have upon the unborn child and avoid recourse to diagnostic procedures which do not offer sufficient guarantees of their honest purpose and substantial harmlessness. And if, as often happens in human choices, a degree of risk must be undertaken, he will take care to assure that it is justified by a truly urgent need for the diagnosis and by the importance of the results that can be achieved by it for the benefit of the unborn child himself" (Pope John Paul II, *Discourse to Participants in the Pro-Life Movement Congress*, December 3, 1982: *Insegnantenti di Giovanni Paolo II*, V, 3 [1982]

when it is done with the thought of possibly inducing an abortion depending upon the results: a diagnosis which shows the existence of a malformation or a hereditary illness must not be the equivalent of a death-sentence. Thus a woman would be committing a gravely illicit act if she were to request such a diagnosis with the deliberate intention of having an abortion should the results confirm the existence of a malformation or abnormality. The spouse or relatives or anyone else would similarly be acting in a manner contrary to the moral law if they were to counsel or impose such a diagnostic procedure on the expectant mother with the same intention of possibly proceeding to an abortion. So too the specialist would be guilty of illicit collaboration if, in conducting the diagnosis and in communicating its results, he were deliberately to contribute to establishing or favoring a link between prenatal diagnosis and abortion.

In conclusion, any directive or program of the civil and health authorities or of scientific organizations which in any way were to favor a link between prenatal diagnosis and abortion, or which were to go as far as directly to induce expectant mothers to submit to prenatal diagnosis planned for the purpose of eliminating fetuses which are affected by malformations or which are carriers of hereditary illness, is to be condemned as a violation of the unborn child's right to life and as an abuse of the prior rights and duties of the spouses.

3. Are therapeutic procedures carried out on the human embryo licit?

As with all medical interventions on patients, *one must uphold as licit procedures carried out on the human embryo which respect the life and integrity of the embryo and do not involve disproportionate risks for it but are directed toward its healing, the improvement of its condition of health, or its individual survival.*

Whatever the type of medical, surgical or other therapy, the free and informed consent of the parents is required, according to the deontological rules followed in the case of children. The application of this moral principle may call for delicate and particular precautions in the case of embryonic or fetal life.

The legitimacy and criteria of such procedures have been clearly stated by Pope John Paul II: "A strictly therapeutic intervention whose explicit objective is the healing of various maladies such as those stemming from chromosomal defects will, in principle, be considered desirable, provided it is directed to the true promotion of the personal well-being of the individual without

---

1512). This clarification concerning "proportionate risk" is also to be kept in mind in the following sections of the present Instruction, whenever this term appears.

doing harm to his integrity or worsening his conditions of life. Such an intervention would indeed fall within the logic of the Christian moral tradition."[28]

4. How is one to evaluate morally research and experimentation* on human embryos and fetuses?

Medical research must refrain from operations on live embryos, unless there is a moral certainty of not causing harm to the life or integrity of the unborn child and the mother, and on condition that the parents have given their free and informed consent to the procedure. It follows that all research, even when limited to the simple observation of the embryo, would become illicit were it to involve risk to the embryo's physical integrity or life by reason of the methods used or the effects induced.

As regards experimentation, and presupposing the general distinction between experimentation for purposes which are not directly therapeutic and experimentation which is clearly therapeutic for the subject himself, in the case in point one must also distinguish between experimentation carried out on embryos which are still alive and experimentation carried out on embryos which are dead. *If the embryos are living, whether viable or not, they must be respected just like any other human person; experimentation on embryos which is not directly therapeutic is illicit.*[29]

No objective, even though noble in itself, such as a foreseeable advantage to science, to other human beings or to society, can in any way justify experimentation on living human embryos or fetuses, whether viable or not, either inside or outside the mother's womb. The informed consent ordinarily required for clinical experimentation on adults cannot be granted by the parents, who may not freely dispose of the physical integrity or life of the unborn

---

* Since the terms "research" and "experimentation" are often used equivalently and ambiguously, it is deemed necessary to specify the exact meaning given them in this document.

1) By *research* is meant any inductive-deductive process which aims at promoting the systematic observation of a given phenomenon in the human field or at verifying a hypothesis arising from previous observations.

2) By *experimentation* is meant any research in which the human being (in the various stages of his existence: embryo, fetus, child or adult) represents the object through which or upon which one intends to verify the effect, at present unknown or not sufficiently known, of a given treatment (e.g. pharmacological, teratogenic, surgical, etc.).

28 Pope John Paul II, *Discourse to the Participants in the 35th General Assembly of the World Medical Association*, October 29, 1983: AAS 76 (1984) 392.

29 Cf. Pope John Paul II, *Address to a Meeting of the Pontifical Academy of Sciences*, October 23, 1982: AAS 75 (1983) 37: "I condemn, in the most explicit and formal way, experimental manipulations of the human embryo, since the human being, from conception to death, cannot be exploited for any purpose whatsoever."

child. Moreover, experimentation on embryos and fetuses always involves risk, and indeed in most cases it involves the certain expectation of harm to their physical integrity or even their death.

To use human embryos or fetuses as the object or instrument of experimentation constitutes a crime against their dignity as human beings having a right to the same respect that is due to the child already born and to every human person. The *Charter of the Rights of the Family* published by the Holy See affirms: "Respect for the dignity of the human being excludes all experimental manipulation or exploitation of the human embryo."[30] The practice of keeping alive human embryos *in vivo* or *in vitro* for experimental or commercial purposes is totally opposed to human dignity.

In the case of experimentation that is clearly therapeutic, namely, when it is a matter of experimental forms of therapy used for the benefit of the embryo itself in a final attempt to save its life, and in the absence of other reliable forms of therapy, recourse to drugs or procedures not yet fully tested can be licit.[31]

The corpses of human embryos and fetuses, whether they have been deliberately aborted or not, must be respected just as the remains of other human beings. In particular, they cannot be subjected to mutilation or to autopsies if their death has not yet been verified and without the consent of the parents or of the mother. Furthermore, the moral requirements must be safeguarded that there be no complicity in deliberate abortion and that the risk of scandal be avoided. Also, in the case of dead fetuses, as for the corpses of adult persons, all commercial trafficking must be considered illicit and should be prohibited.

5. How is one to evaluate morally the use for research purposes of embryos obtained by *in vitro* fertilization?

Human embryos obtained *in vitro* are human beings and subjects with rights: their dignity and right to life must be respected from the first moment of their existence. *It is immoral to produce human embryos destined to be exploited as disposable "biological material."*

---

30 Holy See, *Charter of the Rights of the Family*, 4b: *L'Osservatore Romano*, November 25, 1983.

31 Cf. Pope John Paul II, *Address to the Participants in the Convention of the Pro-Life Movement*, December 3, 1982: *Insegnamenti di Giovanni Paolo II*, V, 3 (1982) 1511: "Any form of experimentation on the fetus that may damage its integrity or worsen its condition is unacceptable, except in the case of a final effort to save it from death." Sacred Congregation for the Doctrine of the Faith, *Declaration on Euthanasia*, 4: AAS 72 (1980) 550: "In the absence of other sufficient remedies, it is permitted, with the patient's consent, to have recourse to the means provided by the most advanced medical techniques, even if these means are still at the experimental stage and are not without a certain risk."

In the usual practice of *in vitro* fertilization, not all of the embryos are transferred to the woman's body; some are destroyed. Just as the Church condemns induced abortion, so she also forbids acts against the life of these human beings. *It is a duty to condemn the particular gravity of the voluntary destruction of human embryos obtained in vitro for the sole purpose of research, either by means of artificial insemination of by means of "twin fission."* By acting in this way the researcher usurps the place of God; and, even though he may be unaware of this, he sets himself up as the master of the destiny of others inasmuch as he arbitrarily chooses whom he will allow to live and whom he will send to death and kills defenseless human beings.

Methods of observation or experimentation which damage or impose grave and disproportionate risks upon embryos obtained *in vitro* are morally illicit for the same reasons. Every human being is to be respected for himself, and cannot be reduced in worth to a pure and simple instrument for the advantage of others. *It is therefore not in conformity with the moral law deliberately to expose to death human embryos obtained in vitro.* In consequence of the fact that they have been produced *in vitro*, those embryos which are not transferred into the body of the mother and are called "spare" are exposed to an absurd fate, with no possibility of their being offered safe means of survival which can be licitly pursued.

6. What judgment should be made on other procedures of manipulating embryos connected with the "techniques of human reproduction"?

Techniques of *in vitro* fertilization can open the way to other forms of biological and genetic manipulation of human embryos, such as attempts or plans for fertilization between human and animal gametes and the gestation of human embryos in the uterus of animals, or the hypothesis or project of constructing artificial uteruses for the human embryo. *These procedures are contrary to the human dignity proper to the embryo, and at the same time they are contrary to the right of every person to be conceived and to be born within marriage and from marriage.*[32] *Also, attempts or hypotheses for obtaining a human being without any connection with sexuality through "twin fission," cloning or parthenogenesis are to be considered contrary to the moral law, since they are in opposition to the dignity both of human procreation and of the conjugal union.*

---

32 No one, before coming into existence, can claim a subjective right to begin to exist; nevertheless, it is legitimate to affirm the right of the child to have a fully human origin through conception in conformity with the personal nature of the human being. Life is a gift that must be bestowed in a manner worthy both of the subject receiving it and of the subjects transmitting it. This statement is to be borne in mind also for what will be explained concerning artificial human procreation.

The freezing of embryos, even when carried out in order to preserve the life of an embryo—cryopreservation—*constitutes an offense against the respect due to human beings* by exposing them to grave risks of death or harm to their physical integrity and depriving them, at least temporarily, of maternal shelter and gestation, thus placing them in a situation in which further offenses and manipulation are possible.

Certain attempts to influence chromosomic or genetic inheritance are not therapeutic but are aimed at producing human beings selected according to sex or other predetermined qualities. These manipulations are contrary to the personal dignity of the human being and his or her integrity and identity. Therefore in no way can they be justified on the grounds of possible beneficial consequences for future humanity.[33] Every person must be respected for himself: in this consists the dignity and right of every human being from his or her beginning.

II. Interventions upon Human Procreation

By "artificial procreation" or "artificial fertilization" are understood here the different technical procedures directed toward obtaining a human conception in a manner other than the sexual union of man and woman. This Instruction deals with fertilization of an ovum in a test-tube (*in vitro* fertilization) and artificial insemination through transfer into the woman's genital tracts of previously collected sperm.

A preliminary point for the moral evaluation of such technical procedures is constituted by the consideration of the circumstances and consequences which those procedures involve in relation to the respect due the human embryo. Development of the practice of *in vitro* fertilization has required innumerable fertilizations and destructions of human embryos. Even today, the usual practice presupposes a hyperovulation on the part of the woman: a number of ova are withdrawn, fertilized and then cultivated *in vitro* for some days. Usually not all are transferred into the genital tracts of the woman; some embryos, generally called "spare," are destroyed or frozen. On occasion, some of the implanted embryos are sacrificed for various eugenic, economic or psychological reasons. Such deliberate destruction of human beings or their utilization for different purposes to the detriment of their integrity and life is contrary to the doctrine on procured abortion already recalled. The connection between *in vitro* fertilization and the voluntary destruction

---

33 Cf. Pope John Paul II, *Discourse to those taking part in the 35th General Assembly of the World Medical Association*, October 29, 1983: AAS 76 (1984) 391.

of human embryos occurs too often. This is significant: through these procedures, with apparently contrary purposes, life and death are subjected to the decision of man, who thus sets himself up as the giver of life and death by decree. This dynamic of violence and domination may remain unnoticed by those very individuals who, in wishing to utilize this procedure, become subject to it themselves. The facts recorded and the cold logic which links them must be taken into consideration for a moral judgment on IVF and ET (*in vitro* fertilization and embryo transfer): the abortion-mentality which has made this procedure possible thus leads, whether one wants it or not, to man's domination over the life and death of his fellow human beings and can lead to a system of radical eugenics.

Nevertheless, such abuses do not exempt one from a further and thorough ethical study of the techniques of artificial procreation considered in themselves, abstracting as far as possible from the destruction of embryos produced *in vitro*.

The present Instruction will therefore take into consideration in the first place the problems posed by heterologous artificial fertilization (II, 1-3),[*] and subsequently those linked with homologous artificial fertilization (II, 4-6).[†]

Before formulating an ethical judgment on each of these procedures, the principles and values which determine the moral evaluation of each of them will be considered.

---

* By the term *heterologous artificial fertilization or procreation*, the Instruction means techniques used to obtain a human conception artificially by the use of gametes coming from at least one donor other than the spouses who are joined in marriage. Such techniques can be of two types:

Heterologous IVF and ET: the technique used to obtain a human conception through the meeting *in vitro* of gametes taken from at least one donor other than the two spouses joined in marriage.

Heterologous artificial insemination: the technique used to obtain a human conception through the transfer into the genital tracts of the woman of the sperm previously collected from a donor other than the husband.

† By *artificial homologous fertilization or procreation*, the Instruction means the technique used to obtain a human conception using the gametes of the two spouses joined in marriage. Homologous artificial fertilization can be carried out by two different methods:

Homologous IVF and ET: the technique used to obtain a human conception through the meeting *in vitro* of the gametes of the spouses joined in marriage.

Homologous artificial insemination: the technique used to obtain a human conception through the transfer into the genital tracts of a married woman of the sperm previously collected from her husband.

A. *Heterologous Artificial Fertilization*

1. Why must human procreation take place in marriage?

Every human being is always to be accepted as a gift and blessing of God. However, from the moral point of view a truly responsible procreation vis-à-vis the unborn child must be the fruit of marriage.

For human procreation has specific characteristics by virtue of the personal dignity of the parents and of the children: the procreation of a new person, whereby the man and the woman collaborate with the power of the Creator, must be the fruit and the sign of the mutual self-giving of the spouses, of their love and of their fidelity.[34] The fidelity of the spouses in the unity of marriage involves reciprocal respect of their right to become a father and a mother only through each other.

The child has the right to be conceived, carried in the womb, brought into the world and brought up within marriage: it is through the secure and recognized relationship to his own parents that the child can discover his own identity and achieve his own proper human development.

The parents find in their child a confirmation and completion of their reciprocal self-giving: the child is the living image of their love, the permanent sign of their conjugal union, the living and indissoluble concrete expression of their paternity and maternity.[35]

By reason of the vocation and social responsibilities of the person, the good of the children and of the parents contributes to the good of civil society; the vitality and stability of society require that children come into the world within a family and that the family be firmly based on marriage.

The tradition of the Church and anthropological reflection recognize in marriage and in its indissoluble unity the only setting worthy of truly responsible procreation.

2. Does heterologous artificial fertilization conform to the dignity of the couple and to the truth of marriage?

Through IVF and ET and heterologous artificial insemination, human conception is achieved through the fusion of gametes of at least one donor other than the spouses who are united in marriage. *Heterologous artificial fertilization is contrary to the unity of marriage, to the dignity of the spouses, to the vocation*

34 Cf. Pastoral Constitution on the Church in the Modern world, *Gaudium et Spes*, no. 50.

35 Cf. Pope John Paul II, Apostolic Exhortation *Familiaris Consortio*, no. 14: AAS 74 (1982) 96.

proper to parents, and to the child's right to be conceived and brought into the world in marriage and from marriage.[36]

Respect for the unity of marriage and for conjugal fidelity demands that the child be conceived in marriage; the bond existing between husband and wife accords the spouses, in an objective and inalienable manner, the exclusive right to become father and mother solely through each other.[37] Recourse to the gametes of a third person, in order to have sperm or ovum available, constitutes a violation of the reciprocal commitment of the spouses and a grave lack in regard to that essential property of marriage which is its unity.

Heterologous artificial fertilization violates the rights of the child; it deprives him of his filial relationship with his parental origins and can hinder the maturing of his personal identity. Furthermore, it offends the common vocation of the spouses who are called to fatherhood and motherhood: it objectively deprives conjugal fruitfulness of its unity and integrity; it brings about and manifests a rupture between genetic parenthood, gestational parenthood and responsibility for upbringing. Such damage to the personal relationships within the family has repercussions on civil society: what threatens the unity and stability of the family is a source of dissension, disorder and injustice in the whole of social life.

These reasons lead to a negative moral judgment concerning heterologous artificial fertilization: consequently fertilization of a married woman with the sperm of a donor different from her husband and fertilization with the husband's sperm of an ovum not coming from his wife are morally illicit. Furthermore, the artificial

---

36 Cf. Pope Pius XII, *Discourse to those taking part in the 4th International Congress of Catholic Doctors*, September 29, 1949: AAS 41 (1949) 559. According to the plan of the Creator, "a man leaves his father and his mother and cleaves to his wife, and they become one flesh" (Gn 2:24). The unity of marriage, bound to the order of creation, is a truth accessible to natural reason. The Church's Tradition and Magisterium frequently make reference to the Book of Genesis, both directly and through the passages of the New Testament that refer to it: Mt 19:4-6; Mk 10:5-8; Eph 5:31. Cf. Athenagoras, *Legatio pro christianis*, 33: PG 6, 965-967; St. Chrysostom, *In Matthaeum homiliae*, LXII, 19, 1: PG 58 597; St. Leo the Great, *Epist. ad Rusticum*, 4: PL 54, 1204; Innocent III, *Epist. Gaudemus in Domino*: DS 778; Council of Lyons II, IV *Session:* DS 860; Council of Trent, XXIV, *Session*: DS 1798. 1802; Pope Leo XIII, Encyclical *Arcanum Divinae Sapientiae*: ASS 12 (1879/80) 388-391; Pope Pius XI, Encyclical *Casti Connubii*: AAS 22 (1930) 546-547; Second Vatican Council, *Gaudium et Spes*, no. 48; Pope John Paul II, Apostolic Exhortation *Familiaris Consortio*, no. 19: AAS 74 (1982) 101-102; *Code of Canon Law*, c.1056.

37 Cf. Pope Pius XII, *Discourse to those taking part in the 4th International Congress of Catholic Doctors*, September 29, 1949: AAS 41 (1949) 560; *Discourse to those taking part in the Congress of the Italian Catholic Union of Midwives*, October 29, 1951: AAS 43 (1951) 850; *Code of Canon Law*, c. 1134.

fertilization of a woman who is unmarried or a widow, whoever the donor may be, cannot be morally justified.

The desire to have a child and the love between spouses who long to obviate a sterility which cannot be overcome in any other way constitute understandable motivations; but subjectively good intentions do not render heterologous artificial fertilization conformable to the objective and inalienable properties of marriage or respectful of the rights of the child and of the spouses.

3. Is "surrogate"* motherhood morally licit?

No, for the same reasons which lead one to reject heterologous artificial fertilization: for it is contrary to the unity of marriage and to the dignity of the procreation of the human person.

Surrogate motherhood represents an objective failure to meet the obligations of maternal love, of conjugal fidelity and of responsible motherhood; it offends the dignity and the right of the child to be conceived, carried in the womb, brought into the world and brought up by his own parents; it sets up, to the detriment of families, a division between the physical, psychological and moral elements which constitute those families.

B. *Homologous Artificial Fertilization*

Since heterologous artificial fertilization has been declared unacceptable, the question arises of how to evaluate morally the process of homologous artificial fertilization: IVF and ET and artificial insemination between husband and wife. First a question of principle must be clarified.

4. What connection is required from the moral point of view between procreation and the conjugal act?

a) The Church's teaching on marriage and human procreation affirms the "inseparable connection, willed by God and unable to be broken by man on

---

* By "surrogate mother" the Instruction means:

a) the woman who carries in pregnancy an embryo implanted in her uterus and who is genetically a stranger to the embryo because it has been obtained through the union of the gametes of "donors." She carries the pregnancy with a pledge to surrender the baby once it is born to the party who commissioned or made the agreement for the pregnancy.

b) the woman who carries in pregnancy an embryo to whose procreation she has contributed the donation of her own ovum, fertilized through insemination with the sperm of a man other than her husband. She carries the pregnancy with a pledge to surrender the child once it is born to the party who commissioned or made the agreement for the pregnancy.

his own initiative, between the two meanings of the conjugal act: the unitive meaning and the procreative meaning. Indeed, by its intimate structure, the conjugal act, while most closely uniting husband and wife, capacitates them for the generation of new lives, according to laws inscribed in the very being of man and of woman."[38] This principle, which is based upon the nature of marriage and the intimate connection of the goods of marriage, has well-known consequences on the level of responsible fatherhood and motherhood. "By safeguarding both these essential aspects, the unitive and the procreative, the conjugal act preserves in its fullness the sense of true mutual love and its ordination toward man's exalted vocation to parenthood."[39]

The same doctrine concerning the link between the meanings of the conjugal act and between the goods of marriage throws light on the moral problem of homologous artificial fertilization, since "it is never permitted to separate these different aspects to such a degree as positively to exclude either the procreative intention or the conjugal relation."[40]

Contraception deliberately deprives the conjugal act of its openness to procreation and in this way brings about a voluntary dissociation of the ends of marriage. Homologous artificial fertilization, in seeking a procreation which is not the fruit of a specific act of conjugal union, objectively effects an analogous separation between the goods and the meanings of marriage.

Thus, *fertilization is licitly sought when it is the result of a "conjugal act which is per se suitable for the generation of children to which marriage is ordered by its nature and by which the spouses become one flesh."*[41] *But from the moral point of view procreation is deprived of its proper perfection when it is not desired as the fruit of the conjugal act, that is to say of the specific act of the spouses' union.*

b) The moral value of the intimate link between the goods of marriage and between the meanings of the conjugal act is based upon the unity of the human being, a unity involving body and spiritual soul.[42] Spouses mutually express their personal love in the "language of the body," which clearly involves both "spousal meanings" and parental ones.[43] The conjugal act by

---

38 Pope Paul VI, Encyclical Letter *Humanae Vitae*, no. 12: AAS 60 (1968) 488-489.

39 *Loc. cit.*, *ibid.*, 489.

40 Pope Pius XII, *Discourse to those taking part in the Second Naples World Congress on Fertility and Human Sterility*, May 19, 1956: AAS 48 (1956) 470.

41 *Code of Canon Law*, c. 1061. According to this Canon, the conjugal act is that by which the marriage is consummated if the couple "have performed (it) between themselves in a human manner."

42 Cf. Pastoral Constitution *Gaudium et Spes*, no. 14.

43 Cf. Pope John Paul II, *General Audience on January 16, 1980: Insegnamenti di Giovanni Paolo II*, III, 1 (1980) 148-152.

which the couple mutually expresses their self-gift at the same time expresses openness to the gift of life. It is an act that is inseparably corporal and spiritual. It is in their bodies and through their bodies that the spouses consummate their marriage and are able to become father and mother. In order to respect the language of their bodies and their natural generosity, the conjugal union must take place with respect for its openness to procreation; and the procreation of a person must be the fruit and the result of married love. The origin of the human being thus follows from a procreation that is "linked to the union, not only biological but also spiritual, of the parents, made one by the bond of marriage."[44] Fertilization achieved outside the bodies of the couple remains by this very fact deprived of the meanings and the values which are expressed in the language of the body and in the union of human persons.

c) Only respect for the link between the meanings of the conjugal act and respect for the unity of the human being make possible procreation in conformity with the dignity of the person. In his unique and unrepeatable origin, the child must be respected and recognized as equal in personal dignity to those who give him life. The human person must be accepted in his parents' act of union and love; the generation of a child must therefore be the fruit of that mutual giving[45] which is realized in the conjugal act wherein the spouses cooperate as servants and not as masters in the work of the Creator who is Love.[46]

In reality, the origin of a human person is the result of an act of giving. The one conceived must be the fruit of his parents' love. He cannot be desired or conceived as the product of an intervention of medical or biological techniques; that would be equivalent to reducing him to an object of scientific technology. No one may subject the coming of a child into the world to conditions of technical efficiency which are to be evaluated according to standards of control and dominion.

The moral relevance of the link between the meanings of the conjugal act and between the goods of marriage, as well as the unity of the human being and the dignity of his origin, demand that the procreation of a human person be brought about as the fruit of the conjugal act specific to the love between spouses. The link between procreation and the conjugal act is thus shown to be of great importance on the anthropological and moral planes, and it throws light on the positions of the Magisterium with regard to homologous artificial fertilization.

---

44 Pope John Paul II, *Discourse to those taking part in the 35th General Assembly of the World Medical Association*, October 29, 1983: AAS 76 (1984) 393.

45 Cf. Pastoral Constitution *Gaudium et Spes*, no. 51.

46 Cf. Pastoral Constitution *Gaudium et Spes*, no. 50.

5. Is homologous *in vitro* fertilization morally licit?

The answer to this question is strictly dependent on the principles just mentioned. Certainly one cannot ignore the legitimate aspirations of sterile couples. For some, recourse to homologous IVF and ET appears to be the only way of fulfilling their sincere desire for a child. The question is asked whether the totality of conjugal life in such situations is not sufficient to ensure the dignity proper to human procreation. It is acknowledged that IVF and ET certainly cannot supply for the absence of sexual relations[47] and cannot be preferred to the specific acts of conjugal union, given the risks involved for the child and the difficulties of the procedure. But it is asked whether, when there is no other way of overcoming the sterility which is a source of suffering, homologous *in vitro* fertilization may not constitute an aid, if not a form of therapy, whereby its moral licitness could be admitted.

The desire for a child—or at the very least an openness to the transmission of life—is a necessary prerequisite from the moral point of view for responsible human procreation. But this good intention is not sufficient for making a positive moral evaluation of *in vitro* fertilization between spouses. The process of IVF and ET must be judged in itself and cannot borrow its definitive moral quality from the totality of conjugal life of which it becomes part nor from the conjugal acts which may precede or follow it.[48]

It has already been recalled that, in the circumstances in which it is regularly practiced, IVF and ET involves the destruction of human beings, which is something contrary to the doctrine on the illicitness of abortion previously mentioned.[49] But even in a situation in which every precaution were taken to avoid the death of human embryos, homologous IVF and ET dissociates from the conjugal act the actions which are directed to human fertilization. For this reason the very nature of homologous IVF and ET also must be taken into account, even abstracting from the link with procured abortion.

Homologous IVF and ET is brought about outside the bodies of the couple through actions of third parties whose competence and technical activity determine the success of the procedure. Such fertilization entrusts the life and identity of the embryo into the power of doctors and biologists and

---

47 Cf. Pope Pius XII, *Discourse to those taking part in the 4th International Congress of Catholic Doctors*, September 29, 1949: AAS 41 (1949) 560: "It would be erroneous . . . to think that the possibility of resorting to this means (artificial fertilization) might render valid a marriage between persons unable to contract it because of the *impedimentum impotentiae*."

48 A similar question was dealt with by Pope Paul VI, Encyclical *Humanae Vitae*, no. 14: AAS 60 (1968) 490-491.

49 Cf. *supra:* I, 1 ff.

establishes the domination of technology over the origin and destiny of the human person. Such a relationship of domination is in itself contrary to the dignity and equality that must be common to parents and children.

Conception *in vitro* is the result of the technical action which presides over fertilization. *Such fertilization is neither in fact achieved nor positively willed as the expression and fruit of a specific act of the conjugal union. In homologous IVF and ET, therefore, even if it is considered in the context of "de facto" existing sexual relations, the generation of the human person is objectively deprived of its proper perfection: namely, that of being the result and fruit of a conjugal act* in which the spouses can become "cooperators with God for giving life to a new person."[50]

These reasons enable us to understand why the act of conjugal love is considered in the teaching of the Church as the only setting worthy of human procreation. For the same reasons the so-called "simple case," i.e., a homologous IVF and ET procedure that is free of any compromise with the abortive practice of destroying embryos and with masturbation, remains a technique which is morally illicit because it deprives human procreation of the dignity which is proper and connatural to it.

Certainly, homologous IVF and ET fertilization is not marked by all that ethical negativity found in extra-conjugal procreation; the family and marriage continue to constitute the setting for the birth and upbringing of the children. Nevertheless, in conformity with the traditional doctrine relating to the goods of marriage and the dignity of the person, *the Church remains opposed from the moral point of view to homologous* in vitro *fertilization. Such fertilization is in itself illicit and in opposition to the dignity of procreation and of the conjugal union, even when everything is done to avoid the death of the human embryo.*

Although the manner in which human conception is achieved with IVF and ET cannot be approved, every child which comes into the world must in any case be accepted as a living gift of the divine Goodness and must be brought up with love.

6. How is homologous artificial insemination to be evaluated from the moral point of view?

Homologous artificial insemination within marriage cannot be admitted except for those cases in which the technical means is not a substitute for the conjugal act but serves to facilitate and to help so that the act attains its natural purpose.

---

50 Pope John Paul II, Apostolic Exhortation *Familiaris Consortio*, no. 14: AAS 74 (1982) 96.

The teaching of the Magisterium on this point has already been stated.[51] This teaching is not just an expression of particular historical circumstances but is based on the Church's doctrine concerning the connection between the conjugal union and procreation and on a consideration of the personal nature of the conjugal act and of human procreation. "In its natural structure, the conjugal act is a personal action, a simultaneous and immediate cooperation on the part of the husband and wife, which by the very nature of the agents and the proper nature of the act is the expression of the mutual gift which, according to the words of Scripture, brings about union 'in one flesh.'"[52] Thus moral conscience "does not necessarily proscribe the use of certain artificial means destined solely either to the facilitating of the natural act or to ensuring that the natural act normally performed achieves its proper end."[53] If the technical means facilitates the conjugal act or helps it to reach its natural objectives, it can be morally acceptable. If, on the other hand, the procedure were to replace the conjugal act, it is morally illicit.

Artificial insemination as a substitute for the conjugal act is prohibited by reason of the voluntarily achieved dissociation of the two meanings of the conjugal act. Masturbation, through which the sperm is normally obtained, is another sign of this dissociation: even when it is done for the purpose of procreation, the act remains deprived of its unitive meaning: "It lacks the sexual relationship called for by the moral order, namely the relationship which realizes 'the full sense of mutual self-giving and human procreation in the context of true love.'"[54]

---

51 Cf. *Response of the Holy Office*, March 17, 1897: DS 3323; Pope Pius XII, *Discourse to those taking part in the 4th International Congress of Catholic Doctors*, September 29, 1949: AAS 41 (1949) 560; *Discourse to the Italian Catholic Union of Midwives*, October 29, 1951: AAS 43 (1951) 850; *Discourse to those taking part in the Second Naples World Congress on Fertility and Human Sterility*, May 19, 1956: AAS 48 (1956) 471-473; *Discourse to those taking part in the 7th International Congress of the International Society of Haematology*, September 12, 1958: AAS 50 (1958) 733; Pope John XXIII, Encyclical *Mater et Magistra*, III: AAS 53 (1961) 447.

52 Pope Pius XII, *Discourse to the Italian Catholic Union of Midwives*, October 29, 1951: AAS 43 (1951) 850.

53 Pope Pius XII, *Discourse to those taking part in the 4th International Congress of Catholic Doctors*, September 29, 1949: AAS 41 (1949) 560.

54 Sacred Congregation for the Doctrine of the Faith, *Declaration on Certain Questions Concerning Sexual Ethics*, 9: AAS 68 (1976) 86, which quotes the Pastoral Constitution *Gaudium et Spes*, no. 51. Cf. *Decree of the Holy Office*, August 2, 1929: AAS 21 (1929) 490; Pope Pius XII, *Discourse to those taking part in the 26th Congress of the Italian Society of Urology*, October 8, 1953: AAS 45 (1953) 678.

7. What moral criterion can be proposed with regard to medical intervention in human procreation?

The medical act must be evaluated not only with reference to its technical dimension but also and above all in relation to its goal which is the good of persons and their bodily and psychological health. The moral criteria for medical intervention in procreation are deduced from the dignity of human persons, of their sexuality and of their origin.

Medicine which seeks to be ordered to the integral good of the person must respect the specifically human values of sexuality.[55] *The doctor is at the service of persons and of human procreation. He does not have the authority to dispose of them or to decide their fate.* A medical intervention respects the dignity of persons when it seeks to assist the conjugal act either in order to facilitate its performance or in order to enable it to achieve its objective once it has been normally performed.[56]

On the other hand, it sometimes happens that a medical procedure technologically replaces the conjugal act in order to obtain a procreation which is neither its result nor its fruit. In this case the medical act is not, as it should be, at the service of conjugal union but rather appropriates to itself the procreative function and thus contradicts the dignity and the inalienable rights of the spouses and of the child to be born.

The humanization of medicine, which is insisted upon today by everyone, requires respect for the integral dignity of the human person first of all in the act and at the moment in which the spouses transmit life to a new person. It is only logical therefore to address an urgent appeal to Catholic doctors and scientists that they bear exemplary witness to the respect due to the human embryo and to the dignity of procreation. The medical and nursing staff of Catholic hospitals and clinics are in a special way urged to do justice to the moral obligations which they have assumed, frequently also, as part of their contract. Those who are in charge of Catholic hospitals and clinics and who are often Religious will take special care to safeguard and promote a diligent observance of the moral norms recalled in the present Instruction.

8. The suffering caused by infertility in marriage

The suffering of spouses who cannot have children or who are afraid of bringing a handicapped child into the world is a suffering that everyone must understand and properly evaluate.

---

55 Cf. Pope John XXIII, Encyclical *Mater et Magistra*, III: AAS 53 (1961) 447.

56 Cf. Pope Pius XII, *Discourse to those taking part in the 4th International Congress of Catholic Doctors*, September 29, 1949: AAS 41 (1949), 560.

On the part of the spouses, the desire for a child is natural: it expresses the vocation to fatherhood and motherhood inscribed in conjugal love. This desire can be even stronger if the couple is affected by sterility which appears incurable. Nevertheless, marriage does not confer upon the spouses the right to have a child, but only the right to perform those natural acts which are *per se* ordered to procreation.[57]

A true and proper right to a child would be contrary to the child's dignity and nature. The child is not an object to which one has a right, nor can he be considered as an object of ownership: rather, a child is a gift, "the supreme gift"[58] *and the most gratuitous gift of marriage, and is a living testimony of the mutual giving of his parents. For this reason, the child has the right, as already mentioned, to be the fruit of the specific act of the conjugal love of his parents; and he also has the right to be respected as a person from the moment of his conception.*

Nevertheless, whatever its cause or prognosis, sterility is certainly a difficult trial. The community of believers is called to shed light upon and support the suffering of those who are unable to fulfill their legitimate aspiration to motherhood and fatherhood. Spouses who find themselves in this sad situation are called to find in it an opportunity for sharing in a particular way in the Lord's Cross, the source of spiritual fruitfulness. Sterile couples must not forget that "even when procreation is not possible, conjugal life does not for this reason lose its value. Physical sterility in fact can be for spouses the occasion for other important services to the life of the human person, for example, adoption, various forms of educational work, and assistance to other families and to poor or handicapped children."[59]

Many researchers are engaged in the fight against sterility. While fully safeguarding the dignity of human procreation, some have achieved results which previously seemed unattainable. Scientists therefore are to be encouraged to continue their research with the aim of preventing the causes of sterility and of being able to remedy them so that sterile couples will be able to procreate in full respect for their own personal dignity and that of the child to be born.

57 Cf. Pope Pius XII, *Discourse to the taking part in the Second Naples World Congress on Fertility and Human Sterility*, May 19, 1956: AAS 48 (1956) 471-473.

58 Pastoral Constitution *Gaudium et Spes*, no. 50.

59 Pope John Paul II, Apostolic Exhortation *Familiaris Consortio*, no. 14: AAS 74 (1982) 97.

III. Moral and Civil Law

The Values and Moral Obligations That Civil Legislation Must Respect and Sanction in This Matter

The inviolable right to life of every innocent human individual and the rights of the family and of the institution of marriage constitute fundamental moral values, because they concern the natural condition and integral vocation of the human person; at the same time they are constitutive elements of civil society and its order.

For this reason the new technological possibilities which have opened up in the field of biomedicine require the intervention of the political authorities and of the legislator, since an uncontrolled application of such techniques could lead to unforeseeable and damaging consequences for civil society. Recourse to the conscience of each individual and to the self-regulation of researchers cannot be sufficient for ensuring respect for personal rights and public order. If the legislator responsible for the common good were not watchful, he could be deprived of his prerogatives by researchers claiming to govern humanity in the name of the biological discoveries and the alleged "improvement" processes which they would draw from those discoveries. "Eugenism" and forms of discrimination between human beings could come to be legitimized: this would constitute an act of violence and a serious offense to the equality, dignity and fundamental rights of the human person.

The intervention of the public authority must be inspired by the rational principles which regulate the relationships between civil law and moral law. The task of the civil law is to ensure the common good of people through the recognition of and the defense of fundamental rights and through the promotion of peace and of public morality.[60] In no sphere of life can the civil law take the place of conscience or dictate norms concerning things which are outside its competence. It must sometimes tolerate, for the sake of public order, things which it cannot forbid without a greater evil resulting. However, the inalienable rights of the person must be recognized and respected by civil society and the political authority. These human rights depend neither on single individuals nor on parents; nor do they represent a concession made by society and the State: they pertain to human nature and are inherent in the person by virtue of the creative act from which the person took his or her origin.

Among such fundamental rights one should mention in this regard: (a) every human being's right to life and physical integrity from the moment of

60 Cf. Declaration *Dignitatis Humanae*, no. 7.

conception until death; (b) the rights of the family and of marriage as an institution and, in this area, the child's right to be conceived, brought into the world and brought up by his parents. To each of these two themes it is necessary here to give some further consideration.

In various States certain laws have authorized the direct suppression of innocents: the moment a positive law deprives a category of human beings of the protection which civil legislation must accord them, the State is denying the equality of all before the law. When the State does not place its power at the service of the rights of each citizen, and in particular of the more vulnerable, the very foundations of a State based on law are undermined. The political authority consequently cannot give approval to the calling of human beings into existence through procedures which would expose them to those very grave risks noted previously. The possible recognition by positive law and the political authorities of techniques of artificial transmission of life and the experimentation connected with it would widen the breach already opened by the legalization of abortion.

As a consequence of the respect and protection which must be ensured for the unborn child from the moment of his conception, the law must provide appropriate penal sanctions for every deliberate violation of the child's rights. The law cannot tolerate—indeed it must expressly forbid—that human beings, even at the embryonic stage, should be treated as objects of experimentation, be mutilated or destroyed with the excuse that they are superfluous or incapable of developing normally.

The political authority is bound to guarantee to the institution of the family, upon which society is based, the juridical protection to which it has a right. From the very fact that it is at the service of people, the political authority must also be at the service of the family.

Civil law cannot grant approval to techniques of artificial procreation which, for the benefit of third parties (doctors, biologists, economic or governmental powers), take away what is a right inherent in the relationship between spouses; and therefore civil law cannot legalize the donation of gametes between persons who are not legitimately united in marriage.

Legislation must also prohibit, by virtue of the support which is due to the family, embryo banks, *post mortem* insemination and "surrogate motherhood."

It is part of the duty of the public authority to ensure that the civil law is regulated according to the fundamental norms of the moral law in matters concerning human rights, human life and the institution of the family. Politicians must commit themselves, through their interventions upon public opinion, to securing in society the widest possible consensus on such essential points and to consolidating this consensus wherever it risks being weakened or is in danger of collapse.

In many countries, the legalization of abortion and juridical tolerance of unmarried couples makes it more difficult to secure respect for the fundamental rights recalled by this Instruction. It is to be hoped that States will not become responsible for aggravating these socially damaging situations of injustice. It is rather to be hoped that nations and States will realize all the cultural, ideological and political implications connected with the techniques of artificial procreation and will find the wisdom and courage necessary for issuing laws which are more just and more respectful of human life and the institution of the family.

The civil legislation of many states confers an undue legitimation upon certain practices in the eyes of many today; it is seen to be incapable of guaranteeing that morality which is in conformity with the natural exigencies of the human person and with the "unwritten laws" etched by the Creator upon the human heart. All men of good will must commit themselves, particularly within their professional field and in the exercise of their civil rights, to ensuring the reform of morally unacceptable civil laws and the correction of illicit practices. In addition, "conscientious objection" vis-à-vis such laws must be supported and recognized. A movement of passive resistance to the legitimation of practices contrary to human life and dignity is beginning to make an ever sharper impression upon the moral conscience of many, especially among specialists in the biomedical sciences.

Conclusion

The spread of technologies of intervention in the processes of human procreation raises very serious moral problems in relation to the respect due to the human being from the moment of conception, to the dignity of the person, of his or her sexuality, and of the transmission of life.

With this Instruction the Congregation for the Doctrine of the Faith, in fulfilling its responsibility to promote and defend the Church's teaching in so serious a matter, addresses a new and heartfelt invitation to all those who, by reason of their role and their commitment, can exercise a positive influence and ensure that, in the family and in society, due respect is accorded to life and love. It addresses this invitation to those responsible for the formation of consciences and of public opinion, to scientists and medical professionals, to jurists and politicians. It hopes that all will understand the incompatibility between recognition of the dignity of the human person and contempt for life and love, between faith in the living God and the claim to decide arbitrarily the origin and fate of a human being.

In particular, the Congregation for the Doctrine of the Faith addresses an invitation with confidence and encouragement to theologians, and above all to moralists, that they study more deeply and make ever more accessible to the faithful the contents of the teaching of the Church's Magisterium in the light of a valid anthropology in the matter of sexuality and marriage and in the context of the necessary interdisciplinary approach. Thus they will make it possible to understand ever more clearly the reasons for and the validity of this teaching. By defending man against the excesses of his own power, the Church of God reminds him of the reasons for his true nobility; only in this way can the possibility of living and loving with that dignity and liberty which derive from respect for the truth be ensured for the men and women of tomorrow. The precise indications which are offered in the present Instruction therefore are not meant to halt the effort of reflection but rather to give it a renewed impulse in unrenounceable fidelity to the teaching of the Church.

In the light of the truth about the gift of human life and in the light of the moral principles which flow from that truth, everyone is invited to act in the area of responsibility proper to each and, like the good Samaritan, to recognize as a neighbor even the littlest among the children of men (cf. Lk 10:29-37). Here Christ's words find a new and particular echo: "What you do to one of the least of my brethren, you do unto me" (Mt 25:40).

During an audience granted to the undersigned Prefect after the plenary session of the Congregation for the Doctrine of the Faith, the Supreme Pontiff, John Paul II, approved this Instruction and ordered it to be published.

Given at Rome, from the Congregation for the Doctrine of the Faith, February 22, 1987, the Feast of the Chair of St. Peter, the Apostle.

Joseph Card. Ratzinger
Prefect

Alberto Bovone
Titular Archbishop of Caesarea in Numidia
Secretary

COMMENTARIES AND STUDIES

A Prophetic Document

MICHEL SCHOOYANS
Professor at the Catholic University of Leuven

The publication of *Donum Vitae* has elicited and increasingly continues to elicit a strong reaction: with her awareness of how similar documents have been received, the Church knows what to expect. However, reactions even stronger than those that followed the publication of *Humane Vitae* are anticipated. That encyclical chiefly addressed the issues of conjugal morality in the strict sense. *Donum Vitae* reiterates and expands on these issues, but it has to do chiefly with new methods, the social, political, and economic repercussions of which are notably significant, and not sufficiently perceived by the public at large. The Instruction does not lose itself in the case studies so dear to certain moralists. It rather consists in a well-made summary document, one that is precise, solidly founded, and not easily ignored.

The key for understanding *Donum Vitae* must be sought in a new and original thesis, preannounced in the title itself. This thesis signals a historic step in the Church's teaching: *one cannot defend human life without at the same time defending the dignity of man, starting with procreation itself.*

The Instruction underscores the essential *link* between these two affirmations. On the one hand, one must defend the life of every human, in every situation, in each of his stages, in his unity of body and soul. On the other hand, one must defend man's dignity. A human being cannot be generated while merely taking the criteria of biological efficacy into account; the baby is not reducible to an "object" over which one has rights; human fecundity has its proper place in the interpersonal cell of the family, united and fruitful, a community of persons, body and soul. What the Church affirms is therefore that respect for human life proceeds in tandem with respect for the conjugal act. *Donum Vitae* starts with man's dignity and the dignity of the couple in judging certain biomedical methods having to do with the transmission of life; it does not start with these latter in order to sell out the respect owed to human life and the family cell.

In reality, at the present moment, we stand before a widespread attitude which is a cause for ever greater disconcertion. On the one hand, there is respect for human life without the respect for human dignity. On this trajectory, we see those who promote the existence of human beings, but these human beings are not necessarily generated in a context that respects the dignity of persons or that of the preborn child. On the other hand, there is the pretense of respecting human dignity but without the respect for life. Thus—leaving sterilization aside for the moment—we see the advocacy for euthanasia, using the justification of wanting to let people "die with dignity." From this point of view the document has no difficulty in showing how the same unholy logic leads to the devaluing of life and the lack of recognition for human dignity.

From the moment in which the force and the coherence of its central thesis is perceived, one realizes that *Donum Vitae* is a prophetic document that will have profound and enduring repercussions.

This prophetic dimension is revealed just by considering the document holistically. Freed from the myopia of case studies, the Instruction invites the Church and the human community to *a long-term perspective*. It asks them to take a moment for reflection. Toward what society are we headed? What society do we wish to build? The document indicates which are dead-end roads, and denounces perversions.

The Church solemnly declares that *all human beings* have the same right to be respected. It therefore decisively opposes the new, subtle forms of eugenics and discrimination. Nor does it even consider a morality of the type that pretends to "legitimize" the elimination of anyone. Thus the Church first of all references the idea of *universality*: all men are equal in rights and in dignity.

The Church also rescues *conjugal union* and the *family* from the destructive devaluation of methods that, though they may be technologically effective, are disastrous for man and for humanity.

Nevertheless, the prophetic dimension of *Donum Vitae* is even more clearly perceptible with regard to the precise points and decisive content having to do with humanity's future.

The Instruction denounces the rupture of the connection between sexuality and procreativity, between "civil" identity and "genetic" identity. The Church opposes this new form of *alienation* that opens the way for the control which the *medical community* wishes to exercise over human life in its origins, over its duration, and over its quality. In particular, the doctor must not appropriate to himself the procreative function of the conjugal act. "In this case the medical act is not, as it should be, at the service of conjugal union but rather appropriates to itself the procreative function and thus contradicts the dignity and the inalienable rights of the spouses and of the child to be born" (II, B, 7).

These dramatic consequences give rise to three possibilities. The first is one in which the doctor would have the authority to "ordain" among different "operations," drawing his power from his elitist knowledge, which legitimizes his "prescriptions." The second is one in which the doctor might be subordinate to powerful private groups, perhaps international groups, who serve to "watch over" the private interests of a minority. The third is one in which the doctor would be a functionary, paid to carry out programs of "social therapy" in which there would be a decrease in the respect owed to persons and to the family.

Thus the Instruction places us on our guard against the emergence of a medical *technocracy*, the ruinous effects of which can already be noted within the context of several societies.

The Instruction is prophetic also in that it reacts against a perversion of *law*, which is almost always connected to the already mentioned perversion of medicine. *Donum Vitae* reminds lawmakers that the law is not utilitarian. As medicine is at the service of human life, so too the law is at the service of justice; it does not exist to promote the interests of the strongest.

In summary, the Instruction is prophetic when it solemnly warns against the degenerations that threaten the doctor and the lawmaker. In other words, this means that medicine and law may become dangerous if they are disconnected from a morality that guarantees human life and its dignity. The human community cannot develop properly once scientific positivism or juridical positivism takes root; nor can it base itself on an individualistic morality, nor on a group morality. In the case of such grave issues it will not do to simply trust the self-regulation of doctors, or of lawmakers, or of politicians—just as, for its part, the morality of business does not merely concern businessmen.

Donum Vitae is also prophetic from the perspective of *Christian morality* in the strict sense. In fact the Instruction does not limit itself to warning against a dehumanizing conception of biomedical discipline. It illuminates how moral problems are to be situated not only on the level of the material elements of the action, but also and above all and prior to all of these, on the level of the intentions and the decisions regarding research.

It is a little simplistic to state that the manufacture of weapons for war is morally indifferent, and to go on to say that the serious moral issues only surface regarding the use to which the weapons will be put. With the research decisions and the techniques that make such weapons available, the researcher anticipates the use that will be made of his discoveries: indeed, he brings about the desire to have recourse to a determinate application that originated from his investigations. One would not proceed with research on nuclear arms were one not united in anticipation with the intention of those who might make use of these arms. And the one who manufactures weapons knows perfectly well for what they will be used.

The same applies to medical research. The moral responsibility of the scientist is involved in advance, with respect to the practical applications that will be derived from his research. He is involved in the decisions we have spoken of by choices that, from the moral perspective, are never neutral or innocent.

The Instruction is prophetic insofar as it points out to the scientist that it is at this fundamental level that he must primarily exercise his "academic freedom." It is at the level of the decisions about research that his moral responsibility is involved, and more so if it is kept in mind that often he is the only one who can foresee the implications of what it is he hopes to discover, and the use to which that discovery can be put.

In brief, there is, certainly, an ethic of the medical profession; but it is sometimes also necessary to underscore that there is an ethic of biomedical research. If medicine wishes to remain at the service of mankind, decisions regarding research must open themselves in a decisive way to the concern for *justice*: there is no morality of pure efficiency. In a world in which, for example, the inequalities surrounding the possibilities of life constitute a scandal that cries to heaven for revenge, morality demands that the priorities of research and of the medical profession be redefined in such a way as fulfills the common good.

In this way, along with the *political* aspect that we have just mentioned, there emerges the final prophetic dimension of *Donum Vitae*. What undergirds the entire document is the strong emphasis on the condition for the possibility of every democracy. *Donum Vitae* goes against the current, but that does not daunt the Church's determination to remain faithful to her mission. The Church *holds today's humanity dear to her heart*, and starting now she holds dear to her heart the humanity of tomorrow. She is concerned for men in places of abundance. She is also concerned for the humanity of the year 2000, four-fifths of whom will live in the Third World. In that moment in which the instruments of domination and the methods of coercion become ever more sophisticated, in that moment in which many men abdicate their liberty in exchange for greater possibilities for their capricious desires, the Church will implore men of good will not to lose sight of what is *essential to their happiness*.

Now what is essential is above all that the right to life, and to a life of dignity, is not the privilege of the king, nor of the nobility, nor of the bourgeoisie, nor of a race of the "elect"; but that it be something belonging to every human being. This dignity is not bestowed or granted by somebody. It is not the result of a vote. It is a truth that impels the intelligence and to which the will adheres by free consent.

It is also essential that we have received this life as a sharing, and it is precisely because of this that we are invited to live it in fraternal communion. Now the ordinary site of this communion, the site in which this personal and inalienable dignity is first recognized, is the family. This is the site *par excellence*, the fundamental site of personalization and socialization, of the gift of self and of the acceptance of the other. The Church teaches us here that the family is the safest defense against individualism and totalitarianism.

The human person will not be saved without saving the family; the family will not be saved without saving the human person. Humanity will not be saved without saving both.

Therefore, from this point of view, which is critical for human society, it must be made manifest from now on that if the Instruction is poorly received, we can be sure that it is because it has been poorly read. It will take at least a generation to recognize that in taking this position, with a courage as serene as it is firm, the Church will have saved man's humanity. At the same time, she is one of those prophets who do not allow themselves to be intimidated: they grit their teeth and sometimes end up at Calvary. But if she were to be silent, the very stones would cry out . . .

The Continuity of the Magisterial Teaching

ANGEL RODRIGUEZ LUÑO
Instructor of Morality at the John Paul II Institute and the Roman Academic Center of Holy Cross

As can be deduced from the title of the recent Instruction of the Congregation for the Doctrine of the Faith, there are at bottom two moral questions that are addressed: the respect for human life in its origin and the dignity of procreation. On both of these issues the document "does not intend to repeat all the Church's teaching," but rather "to offer, in the light of the previous teaching of the Magisterium," concrete answers to certain specific problems emerging from the field of biomedicine.

The role played by the preceding Magisterium's doctrine with respect to both the moral judgments here contained and their justification, is rather evident from the footnotes with which the Instruction is furnished. Nonetheless, as is called for in the case of this kind of document, which was chosen by the Congregation, the notes and citations inspire a certain sobriety. It has therefore seemed to me not wholly superfluous to launch a theological reflection on the magisterial supports of the present Instruction.

1. The first issue to be examined is that of the respect owed to human embryos. The introductory statement, "The human being must be respected—as a person—from the very first instant of his existence" (I, 1), reasserts the moral criterion, one universally accepted since the earliest times, of Tradition and of the Church's Magisterium. It would be useless to tarry in order to prove this. The Instruction explicitly cites the *Declaration on Procured Abortion*, which provided brief but complete information about the principal witnesses of the Tradition, beginning with the *Didache* or *The Teaching of the Twelve Apostles* (ca. 90-100), and of the principle documents of the Magisterium.

It is a doctrine that, in the words of Pope Paul VI, has not changed and is unchangeable. Today many authors converge in thinking that, in light of the Dogmatic Constitution *Lumen Gentium* (nos. 12 and 25), there exist all the conditions needed to state that the inviolability of human life from the precise moment of conception is *a moral truth infallibly professed and taught by the Church* (cf., for example, L. Ciccone, *Non uccidere*, Ares, Milano, 1984, pp. 28-40). It is moreover traditionally the conviction that, as far as concerns the moral attitude to be held, the theoretical discussions surrounding the moment of the spiritual soul's infusion are not substantially determinative. I will not reference the words of Athenagoras and Tertullian, which everyone knows at this point. Even St. Basil, in condemning abortion, displays the same persuasion when he admonishes, "Let us not quibble among ourselves over whether the fetus is formed or not" (*Letters*, 188, 2 [To Amphilochius], in the year 374).

Nevertheless it seems clear to me that the present Instruction, while reiterating that "the Magisterium has not expressly committed itself to an affirmation of a philosophical nature" (I, 1), takes into account the fact that recent scientific findings offer indications "for discerning by the use of reason a personal presence at the moment of this first appearance of a human life" (I, 1). Perhaps this is why it speaks not only of the respect owed to human life, but rather that "the human being must be respected—as a person" (I, 1), and affirms that embryos "must be respected just like any other human person" (I, 4): such statements, within their context, seek to establish a practical criterion, but they become significant precisely because they are not required to define a norm of behavior.

2. The second moral issue is that of the dignity of human procreation, relative to the techniques of artificial procreation (artificial insemination, *in vitro* fertilization followed by the transferal of the embryo). The Magisterium's prior teaching is presented, as a general principle, in the Introduction: "Human procreation requires on the part of the spouses responsible collaboration with the fruitful love of God (cf. *Gaudium et Spes*, no. 50); the gift of human life must be actualized in marriage through the specific and exclusive acts of husband and wife, in accordance with the laws inscribed in their persons and in their union (cf. *Gaudium et Spes*, no. 51)" (Introduction, 5), and these laws are, as Pope John XXIII stated, most holy, immutable, and inviolable (cf. Introduction, 4, in which *Mater et Magistra* is cited).

I maintain that these laws are to be considered most holy and immutable, not merely because they are uncontrived; rather they are most holy and immutable because they alone correspond to God's designs, which we know through biblical sources ("Have you not read that from the beginning the Creator . . ." (Mt 19:4-6), and because they alone define the exercise of the sexuality that is proper to marriage, to that sacrament that "*from the beginning* has be constituted in the sign of the *union of flesh*" (Pope John Paul II, *Catecheses on Human Love*, August 22, 1984).

In the light of the Catholic doctrine on marriage, there can be no doubt about the negative evaluation of artificial heterologous procreation (outside of marriage or contrary to marriage), nor about the reasons for this moral judgment. As to the concrete judgment formulated by Pius XII, in absolute terms, this judgment cannot be characterized as having a limited or circumstantial worth, since it is based on the unity of marriage, which carries with it a right-obligation "to become a father and a mother only through each other" (II, A, 1). The unity of marriage brings about, according to God the Creator's designs, a bond that is even stronger than that uniting parents and children: "A man leaves his father and mother and clings to his wife, and the two of them become one body" (Gn 2:24; for the magisterial teaching on this point, cf. footnote 36 of the Instruction). When offspring are only possible by means of interventions detrimental to the unity of marriage, the desire for children is no longer the desire for a good, and thus it loses its natural righteousness; "it is better and more just to die without children than to procure offspring through an illicit union" (St. Augustine, *On the Good of Marriage*, c. 16, no. 18; cf. ibid., c. 14, no. 16; c. 24, no. 32 and *On the Literal Meaning of Genesis*, book IX, c. 7, no. 12).

3. The Instruction expresses a negative moral judgment also when confronting homologous artificial procreation, the reasons for which are summarized with the following words: "*The moral relevance of the link between the meanings of the conjugal act and between the goods of marriage, as well as the unity of the human being and the dignity of his origin, demand that the procreation of a human person be brought about as the fruit of the conjugal act specific to the love between spouses*. The link between procreation and the conjugal act is thus shown to be of great importance on the anthropological and moral planes, and it throws light on the positions of the Magisterium with regard to homologous artificial fertilization" (II, B, 4).

As far as IVF and ET, the judgment also covers the so-called "simple case," that is, a procedure of *in vitro* fertilization, "free of any compromise with the abortive practice of destroying embryos and with masturbation" (II, B, 5), since in every case IVF and ET "dissociates from the conjugal act the actions which are directed to human fertilization" (II, B, 5). A similar declaration makes it superfluous to spend much time here by reviewing the circumstance that "the connection between *in vitro* fertilization and the voluntary destruction of human embryos occurs too often" (II). This is a very relevant fact, primarily because, in its own way, it demonstrates that there is no better protection of new life than that guaranteed by the intimacy of conjugal love; in other words, this a not-insignificant aspect of the value belonging to the connection between conjugal union and procreation, of which more will be said later.

In order to expound more fully the reason for the moral criterion given by the Instruction, it will be appropriate to restate a principle that has already been expressed. It would be difficult to maintain that the satisfaction of any desire always constitutes a good. We have all been exposed to the test of irrational desires. Certainly, the desire for offspring is not irrational, but in certain conditions it might become so. What are such conditions? Certainly not those propagandized by Neo-Malthusianism; the Church has always held that *the event of a human being's generation* is a good, provided that it is in keeping with the fuller good that naturally contains it. From St. Augustine onward, this fuller good has been called the good of marriage, which has three parts (*tripartitum est*); the three parts have been given the names *fides*, *proles*, *et sacramentum* (cf. St. Augustine, *On the Literal Meaning of Genesis*, book IX, c. 7, no. 12). Often in the documents of the Magisterium the same concept is presented with a different expression: the language used is that of connection. Thus Pope Pius XI states, "Every sin committed as regards the offspring becomes in some way a sin against conjugal faith, since both these blessings are essentially connected" (Encyclical Letter *Casti Connubii*, December 31, 1930: AAS 22 [1930] 565-566.

In the more recent Magisterium there has indubitably been a theological deepening regarding the nature and ethical worth of this connection. In this area it seems effort is needed to reach a more exact definition than that which was traditionally called *bonum fidei*.

Fides is not exclusively fidelity between the spouses: fidelity is a consequence of the fact that belongs to the very nature of marriage as an official act, or even an institutional act, of reciprocal, total, exclusive, and definitive giving between the spouses; an act that is certainly vivified by conjugal love. *Fides* belongs, according to St. Thomas, to the constitutive structure of marriage (cf. *Summa Theologiae*, III, q. 29, a. 3, c) and is hence prior to the acts by which the ends are reached: mutual giving is not an end; rather it should be said that the generation of offspring and the mutual aid are the ends—the reason for being—of the conjugal giving and therefore of the marriage. Perhaps it is necessary to state that the mutual giving, vivified by conjugal love, is a dynamic principle, which is therefore endowed with an intrinsic orientation to certain ends. As long as this aspect remained unappreciated, theological advancement regarding the nature of *fides* was torturous and difficult, because it involved implications that may have seemed to many—and not without reason—to be misleading: indeed, emphatically underscoring the theological and anthropological importance and profundity of something that was erroneously placed with the ends was like defending the moral self-sufficiency of this "second end," which would have overshadowed—against the Church's entire tradition—the worth of procreation.

The terminology of the pastoral Constitution *Gaudium et Spes* dissolved every equivocation (cf., for example, nos. 48:1; 49:2; 50:1. See too F. Gil Hellin, "Los 'bona matrimonii' en la Constitución pastoral *Gaudium et Spes*": *Scripta Theologica* 11 [1979] 127-176). Conjugal union has two values and two significant meanings: the unitive meaning, which expresses and consummates the very nature of marriage as mutual giving, vivified by conjugal love; and the procreative meaning, which corresponds to the primary and essential finality of matrimony. It is only with respect for both meanings that one can speak of a truly conjugal or matrimonial exercise of sexuality. Very important in this regard is *Gaudium et Spes*'s reference to "the objective . . . criteria drawn from the nature of the human person and human action, *criteria which respect the total meaning of mutual self-giving and human procreation in the context of true love*" (*Donum Vitae*, n22, [emphasis added]).

At this point, the following question arises: Does it necessarily follow from this criterion that both meanings must be present together in every single act, even when, for reasons not traceable to the will of the spouses, such is neither easy nor possible? We need not here engage in a study of the history of the text of number 51 of *Gaudium et Spes*, nor of the particular circumstances in which it was developed. As is well-known, the footnote added to the text to indicate the existence of a special commission to study the issues of population, of family, and of birthrate, directs us to look for an answer in the Encyclical *Humanae Vitae*, and specifically in paragraph number 12. Indeed, the necessity that every individual conjugal act must remain open to the transmission of life is based "on the inseparable connection, established by God, which man on his own initiative may not break, between the unitive significance and the procreative significance which are both inherent to the marriage act."

That the value of this connection must also support the moral judgment on artificial fertilization, including *in vitro*, was already affirmed by Pope Pius XII (cf. II, B, 4, footnote 40, and II, B, 6, footnote 51). The Instruction makes it clear that the moral criterion formulated by Pope Pius XII and by Pope John XXII "is based on the Church's doctrine concerning the connection between the conjugal union and procreation and on a consideration of the personal nature of the conjugal act and of human procreation" (II, B, 6). As I see it, the Pastoral Constitution *Gaudium et Spes*, the Encyclical *Humanae Vitae*, and the Apostolic Exhortation *Familiaris Consortio* (cf. nos. 11-12; 14-15; 18-20; and 28-32) have made this reasoning more understandable, since they have clearly expounded the reasons according to which the connection between the unitive and procreative aspect of sexuality is what defines, in an exclusive way, the truly conjugal realization of human sexuality. That sexuality is truly conjugal that faithfully and integrally expresses the nature (and hence the good) of marriage: the spouses' reciprocal, total, and definitive gift, which has as its chief reason for existing the cooperation with God in the transmission of human life. The spouses carry out this mutual gift in their "unified totality" (cf. *Familiaris Consortio*, no. 11) and so also carry it out according to the language of the body, which makes of them one flesh. "*Fertilization is licitly sought when it is the result of a 'conjugal act which is per se suitable for the generation of children to which marriage is ordered by its nature and by which the spouses become one flesh'* (*Code of Canon Law*, c. 1061)" (II, B, 4).

Why need this be the case? The answer is simple. According to the moral norm that has always existed in the Church, the unique legitimate realization of sexuality is conjugal or matrimonial. Consequently the present Instruction appears in harmony and in continuity with the developments of the most recent Magisterium on the exact meaning that *fides*—which is really conjugal communion in its physical, psychological, and spiritual dimensions—assumes in the theology of matrimony. The document in question demonstrates that neither homologous artificial insemination nor homologous *in vitro* fertilization objectively constitute a conjugal or matrimonial realization of sexuality, just as other sexual behaviors between a couple, behaviors that are not detrimental to the *bonum prolis*, may also fail to constitute a conjugal or matrimonial realization of sexuality (cf. *Humanae Vitae*, no. 13): these latter neither realize nor express the spiritual aspects of conjugal communion, just as homologous artificial procreation neither realizes nor expresses the physical aspect ("one flesh"). Only those acts which are sure to "respect the total meaning of mutual self-giving and human procreation in the context of true love" (*Gaudium et Spes*, no. 51, cited in *Donum Vitae*, n22) are truly conjugal—"acts which are properly spousal."

This summons to conjugal communion can clarify the meaning of that reference to the dignity and to the rights of the human being who is yet to be born. The person's dignity requires above all that he be considered a person and treated as such: that is, it is necessary that one have toward him a loving attachment (which is the precept of charity!), excluding thereby any utilitarian mindset from the interpersonal relationship. By means of the dynamic intrinsic to the acts proper to the spouses, procreation remains objectively immersed—we may prescind from the possible privations of individual persons—in a context of true love, but the same cannot be said of artificial procreation.

Clearly we are not speaking here of the subjective intentions of the spouses, since these cannot inherently either determine or change the logic proper to a technical process. We are speaking of the requirements that are linked to clinical methods, which we can become familiar with through the main international specialized magazines. It might be thought that techniques will improve and that their cost in human life will decrease; we might even admit as much. But from a moral point of view, the crucial fact is that while the human cost is high—it is today and it was even more so in the past—*these techniques have been applied without any manner of scruple*. Objectively, the motive is not respect for the person, since "to not respect today" in order "to maybe respect tomorrow" is a contradictory attitude, and thinking that "not respecting today" might result in "respecting in the future" is equally incongruous. This simple reflection should lead us to understand that the demand underlying the present Instruction is that of reiterating that the dignity of the person constitutes a boundary beyond which one must not go: perhaps some desires will remain unsatisfied, but it is indubitably certain that the progress of medicine at the service of the human person will not be hindered.

Science and Morality

BARTHOLOMEW KIELY, SJ
Gregorian Pontifical University

1. Progress in the biological and medical sciences gives rise (more directly than progress in other areas of natural science) to moral questions, and science as such cannot give adequate answers to these questions. This point will be developed briefly in the following paragraphs, in the hope of providing an initial orientation to the reading of the recent Instruction. It is in no way intended as a devaluation of biology or medicine. A short time spent working in a laboratory is enough to learn how much labor is needed for even minor discoveries; and any illness whatsoever will remind us how much we owe to modern medicine. But the fact remains that new biomedical techniques involve new powers over human life; responsibility goes with power; and such responsibility must be guided by norms based on the respect due to the human person.

2. When an action is described in general and abstract terms, without specifying who acts and who undergoes the action, it is easy to lose sight of important aspects of its moral quality; for the action can have very different meanings for the person who performs it and for the person who undergoes it. (Some current expressions, as when abortion is called "the interruption of pregnancy," are chosen precisely in order to avoid attracting attention to this aspect of the problem; after all, the idea of interrupting an abstraction does not invite the kind of reaction that would be provoked by another description of the same reality.) Progress in biology and medicine gives new powers to *some people* over *other people*; these powers may be used for good or for ill; and they require in any case a moral orientation.

3. As to the application of these new techniques, let us consider first the person who is active. Anyone able to carry out such a procedure must, with a certain inevitability, be a privileged person; already an adult, more intelligent than most, and having a role that is respected by society. The rights of such a person will be secure; adults who are highly trained are in general respected. Such a person possesses certain real powers, since he can carry out difficult tasks that are beyond the abilities of most people; science, especially practical

science, is a recognized form of power. In brief, such a scientist is a person who is privileged in our society and has no special reason to fear a violation of his own rights.

Furthermore, the scientist possesses a symbolic kind of power, as a representative (one might say a priest or even prelate) of a contemporary form of implicit religion, namely, technology. For technology has, for many people at the present time, a status that is in effect religious, as the basis of an *ultimate* hope for the future of humanity. It seems to inspire great reverence, to the point of superstition, perhaps especially in those who know it from a distance, never having actually worked in a laboratory. So science can be, for some and perhaps for many, a kind of contemporary idol; and it seems to me that some negative reactions to the Instruction will arise from this very point, in the sense that some people may feel that the supreme and practically sacred value of technical progress has been insulted.

4. But we must also remember the person who undergoes the application of any technique; and this point brings us to the center of the problem. Sometimes the rights of this person are more obvious, but at other times less so. When a person is in the years of his maturity, his physical qualities give clear expression to his worth as a person; the person himself and his relatives are more able and willing to defend his rights, including the right to life and to bodily integrity. Accordingly, society gives relatively good protection to these rights; one may recall, for example, the many tests and trials that a new medicine must go through before it can be sold to the public. When somebody has reached the last stages of his earthly life, or is severely handicapped, his physical condition corresponds less clearly to his value as a person; and here arise the problems of euthanasia. These problems, for all their importance, are not part of this article. The immediately relevant point is that an aged person is still a powerful symbol, having a form that is clearly human; and even a human corpse inspires reverence. But the problem in question becomes especially acute when the human being does not yet have a visible form that is obviously human. The sight of a newborn child, who already appears human, arouses a moral emotion which makes his life effectively sacred; practically nobody would wish to justify infanticide. Once the face of the baby has been seen, it becomes psychologically impossible to kill it. But a fetus does not have the same power over our emotions, since its face has never been seen. The commonly accepted distinction between infanticide and abortion seems to be based far more on emotional reactions to symbols (especially to the powerful symbol that is the face of a baby) than on moral reasoning. Yet the fetus, even after a few months of gestation, has an external form that is clearly human (if only it could be seen); and there exists a body

of psychiatric research indicating that the woman who aborts without much regret has repressed the normal process of symbolic fantasy about the fetus she is carrying.

This problem (namely, that our first moral reactions depend on the symbolic qualities of the object) becomes even more important when we are dealing with human life in its origin. Each of us (we should remember) has had a very humble beginning as a microorganism, a single cell (zygote) whose external form was not so very different from that of a common amoeba. But science has shown that the human zygote is one of the wonders of nature, perhaps the greatest of all in terms of its level of organization. It already contains in its nucleus the complete genetic program of the mature human body, a program equivalent to more than a thousand megabytes packed into a microscopic space. This program seems remarkably economic, given the complexity of the mature body, which has a brain containing a thousand million neurons, each as complex as a small computer. As the embryo grows to a fetus, the formation of different tissues involves a process of *self*-selection carried out by the initial genetic program, so that in each kind of cell some parts of the program are operative and others are suppressed. Each differentiated cell is then rather like a child that was born knowing all the branches of science, but who later became a specialist by forgetting all disciplines save one. When conception has occurred, the genetic program is already complete; and if there were a question of copyright on the program, it would have to be recognized from that moment, precisely because the basic "text" is already complete. The fact of spontaneous twinning raises some philosophical problems, but these are not insoluble; and the fact remains that the zygote need only be left alone in order to develop into a baby. The very fact that the embryo can carry out the early stages of its development *in vitro* confirms that a *new* human life has begun and is already under its own management. These facts are matched by the teaching of *Gaudium et Spes*, number 51, that "from the moment of conception life must be guarded with the greatest care." Besides, in the light of faith we grasp the point that the conception of a new life is a more solemn event than a sentence of death; the new life is eternal, while death is only a kind of transition.

But the fact remains that the human zygote or embryo does not appeal greatly to our imagination and emotions; its force as a symbol is limited. It is therefore particularly exposed to the danger of becoming a victim of the new powers of technicians over human life.

5. In such a context has appeared the recent Instruction on the respect due to human life in its origin and to the dignity of procreation; to uphold the rights of the defenseless, to uphold at the very beginnings of life the

protection due to the human person, and further to point out that this kind of respect means that the child must be born as the fruit of the incarnate love of two parents who are married to each other, a love expressed in a way that is specific to, and reserved to, marriage.

New human lives are defended against the manipulation of embryos, and especially against experimentation on what are called "spare embryos," those that are not destined to be implanted into the body of a mother.

The origin of life is also defended against ways of procreating that are not in keeping with the value of the new life that is coming to be; ways that involve a technical domination over life, as when fertilization takes place *in vitro*. Such techniques really do involve a relationship of domination and subjection, and really do treat the new human being as a subhuman thing, placed in a position of inevitable inferiority. (I believe that anyone who has ever carried out a laboratory experiment can grasp this point; one's attitude to a piece of apparatus or to the contents of a test tube is very different from the attitude one has to another human person.) The situation is quite different when two spouses give sexual expression to their love, being ready to accept a child as a free gift from God; in so doing, they do not place a new life on a level of inferiority with respect to themselves.

6. The teaching of this Instruction is based above all on various aspects of *unity* in human life: the unity of the person as embodied spirit, which means that the body shares fully in the value of the person, both in the life of the individual and also in the procreation of new life. The teaching of this Instruction is also based on the inseparable connection between the two meanings of the marriage act, the unitive and the procreative. With regard to this unity, it may be noted that the unity of two meanings, in contrast to the unity of two material things or processes, suggests that both meanings form part of a single meaning at a deeper level. It may be (as suggested by Robert Barry and Francis X. Meehan) that the only analogy that does justice to this deeper meaning is to be found in the Blessed Trinity, in which union and generation coincide perfectly. It is also worth noting that the explanation of a unity is inevitably difficult, since an explanation has to proceed by taking one aspect at a time, making it easy to lose sight of the unity that is the whole point of the explanation. (One meets a somewhat similar difficulty when the point of a joke has to be explained.) On the other hand, it would be all too easy, as a controversial tactic, to prescind from the unity that is the most basic issue, and dispute the Instruction part by part.

7. In such terms one can see that the Instruction is not superfluous, nor is it an unjustified invasion of the territory of science on the part of the Magisterium. We should not forget that the principle that all persons

are fundamentally equal, just because they are human persons, has become widely accepted in philosophy, thanks also to the labors of Kant. But this principle was not fully evident either to Plato or to Aristotle, nor is it evident to many of our contemporaries; so it is not really a principle simply to be taken for granted. The justification of this principle given in *Gaudium et Spes* (no. 29) is theological, not philosophical. A failure to grasp this principle can be seen especially in the widespread practice of abortion; it is very difficult to doubt that a fetus, after ten weeks (say) of gestation, is a human being (its human status being by this point more immediately *obvious* in comparison to the situation of the zygote); and yet there are doctors who practice abortion without scruple. This very point also goes to show that a mastery of medical techniques by no means guarantees that a doctor or scientist will have a moral sense, or a moral training, that is at the same level as his professional skills. In fact, going by my own experience as a biochemist, and as someone who was reared in a family of Catholic surgeons, it seems that the categories and methods of *formal* moral reasoning are difficult for anyone who has not had a special training in the area, even for someone who is highly intelligent and has profound moral *intuitions*. Even people who accept *Humanae Vitae* do not seem to come to a full grasp of its meaning and logic. They can see in an intuitive way that artificial contraception opens the way to selfishness and related abuses; but it is hard for them to get much beyond that level. Obviously enough, to grasp an argument based on the integral worth of the human person (even when life is in its earliest phases) will be much more difficult for doctors or scientists who are not believers.

One must therefore foresee as inevitable some refusals to accept this Instruction. The contemporary world rejects other teachings of the Church, on divorce and abortion, for example. But that does not mean that these teachings are false or outdated.

Opposition from some moralists is also to be anticipated. An approach that is widespread in contemporary Catholic moral thinking would base the evaluation of human actions, in part or totally, on the balance of their positive and negative consequences. This kind of approach in effect shares the technological outlook, and represents a morality that is teleological in an *extrinsic* or utilitarian sense; it is focused on the results that are hoped for, attributing moral significance mainly or solely to the intention of the agent, but not to the intelligible form of the actions themselves. An approach to morality that has in effect adopted the technological outlook is not in a position to criticize this outlook when a critique is necessary. The anthropological approach of the Instruction is different (as is that of the preceding teaching of the Magisterium on which it draws) and represents an *intrinsic* teleology focused on the inherent meaning of a given way of acting and its correspondence, or lack of correspondence, with the integral vocation and worth of the human person, whether of the person who acts, or of the person who undergoes the action.

In a utopia, in which everyone had a deep appreciation of the value of every human person at every stage of the person's life, this Instruction would have been less necessary. But we are not living in any such utopia. We must also remember that, quite probably, we are still in the early stages of a phase of accelerating technical development, whose limits nobody can foresee. Perhaps the twentieth century will be referred to by future historians as the "paleotechnical period." So we live at a time in which the defense of the values of family life is particularly important. If the Church does not undertake this defense, who can be expected to do so? (One may recall the timidity with which health authorities seem to suggest the possibility of monogamy as a defense against the spread of AIDS.)

It is therefore a duty of particular urgency to defend the conditions of human life and its transmission, not only at the level of the person's interiority, but also as to the physical conditions of life and of procreation. This requirement corresponds to the strange nature of the human person as the animal made in the image and likeness of God: the animal who is eternal.

The Theological Principle of Human Procreation

ANGELO SCOLA
John Paul II Institute
Pontifical Lateran University

1. Separate procreation from sexuality; that way you can control the process and the fruit of the first and reduce the second to pure pleasure! Based on the "dominant ideology" (cf. the Instruction *Donum Vitae*, Introduction, 2), this might seem to be the final objective of biomedical science's shocking pursuits. Motivations, goals, and means of a project like this then underlie an indefinite possibility of variations that, when closely scrutinized, are such as to make even the most daring science fiction pale by comparison.

Even among unbelievers, there are not a few persons who fear the possible outcomes of such a "biogenetic revolution," which might lead man to the threshold of an apocalypse no less grave than a nuclear one. Nonetheless, it is said, science and technology *must* march onward, as though this were the requirement of some *higher decree*, which one may never legitimately fail to observe. Naturally, some of the more "meritorious" reasons for this undertaking are highlighted, those that seek, with human compassion, to attend to the "suffering of spouses who cannot have children or who are afraid of bringing a handicapped child into the world" (II, 8). If someone dares raise his voice to question the reasons for such a technological imperative, or wonders about the anthropological "fittingness" of this project, effort is made to portray him as an obscurantist, one insensitive to the pain of so many couples.

In this context, the Instruction *Donum Vitae* prophetically resounds with the voice of freedom, full of courage, in appealing to all men of today, both believers and nonbelievers, to understand the authentic sense of what is at stake in the astounding possibility of biomedical science. And this it does by once again drawing an extraordinary energy from the inexhaustible heritage of the Church's tradition, energy capable of illuminating, in its different facets, humanity's present and future. It is the light of Christ, who with the Incarnation unites himself in some way to every man (cf. *Gaudium et Spes*, no. 22) and allows everyone to better see the light of God's face impressed upon one's own heart (cf. Ps 4:7). It was with this verse from the Psalms that Thomas documented the existence of man's natural law.

2. The project of separating procreation from sexuality sacrifices the authentic meaning of human sexuality. It is in fact relegated to the inter-cosmic, at the level of any other animal sexuality. And yet human sexuality has been destined for something quite different! It is a constitutive part of man's being in the image of God; "in the image of God he created them; / male and female he created them!" (Gn 1:27b). This is a position maintained, with different emphases, by Barth, by Przywara, and by Balthasar. The first Genesis story, attributed to the priestly source, appears to be characterized by an ascending narrative structure in that it describes an ascending generative outlook. It in fact portrays beings as emerging in an order of increasing dignity by God's creative decree. And when man appears, the narrative introduces the idea that is incessantly reprised by the great Catholic tradition, that of God's image. Thus sexuality appears as an original fact in the human creature, as is also suggested by the evidence of man's constitution, contrary to every temptation to present it as an effect of Original Sin.

This view of things establishes a radical difference between man and the other animals, between human and animal sexuality.

What then is the ultimate meaning of human sexuality? We must try to go deeper in our understanding of the Creator-creature relationship, as expressed by the idea of the *imago Dei*.

We know that creation comes from the Trinitarian God. Thomas and Bonaventure, each with different areas of emphasis, insist on affirming the decisive importance of the Trinitarian principle in creation. "Since inequalities emerge from equalities" (*Hexaemeron* XI, 9), the eternal processions in God constitute the *principle of order* (*ratio ordinis*) of the procession of creatures from God (cf. *Summa Theologiae*, I, q. 45, a. 6). Due to the intervention of the divine Persons in the creative act, creatures bear the imprint of the *imago Trinitatis*. In the intra-Trinitarian relationship, the Father communicates to the Son the very essence of his divinity, such that the Son's whole being is in relationship with the thought and will of the Father. The love that is established between the two co-spirates the Holy Spirit, who is the overflowing seal of the inexhaustible love that unites Father and Son. Man, destined to be a son in the Son, is for this reason created in God's image; he realizes in all the dimensions of his being, which is *corpore et anima unus* (*Gaudium et Spes*, no. 4), the "form" impressed by the Creator. Only in an attitude of creaturely humility can man live out his being as an image of God. The creative act that makes him to be in this way actually suspends him in a double-distance between his Creator and nothingness. If man forgets this, he will self-destruct.

Such a state of affairs also impacts the profound nature of human sexuality. Precisely because God's love is doubly fecund—in an intra-Trinitarian manner in the very Person of the Spirit, and in an extra-Trinitarian manner in creation—so too is human love, insofar as created love participates in this profound dynamism, constitutive of being, which is fecundity. Human love essentially implies fertility. This is why fertility is inscribed within the nature of human sexuality. In the exercise of his sexuality man cannot leave aside this structural openness to procreation at the expense of closing himself to God's creative initiative, the same initiative that impresses upon the heart the seal of Trinitarian fruitfulness.

3. Without going over all the passages, it is this understanding of things that makes human fruitfulness dependent on Trinitarian fruitfulness, based on human sexuality's original state of belonging to the *imago Dei*. The very nature of sexual reciprocity prevents all this from seeming abstract. From the first, the mystery of man is securely placed in reference to the image corresponding to him—namely, the woman—and vice versa. The second creation narrative, that of the Yahwist, very nicely underscores this fact of being made, one for the other: "This one, at last, is bone of my bones / and flesh of my flesh" (Gn 2:23). Nonetheless, man may not exert any domination over the woman, as he is called to do instead over all the other *animals*. Though by their sexuality they are structurally made for each other, they are exposed to a permanent, *irreducible* difference. In this way sexual difference emerges as an ineradicable fact, and, from within the one human nature, man is constituted as a *dual reality*. Contrary to the imaginative thesis expressed by Aristophanes in Plato's *Symposium*, no sexual union can eliminate, in an impossible, definitive fulfillment, that radical difference that is the difference between the sexes.

The dialectical structure of sexual reciprocity is in itself one of the signs of the creature's contingency, but we are here concerned to emphasize a different aspect, one more pertinent to the present theme. That sexual union cannot bring about the elimination of the difference between man and woman depends on the fact that it is metaphysically open to the generation *of another human*. It is the intrinsic orientation of sexuality to procreation that reveals the whole meaning of sexual reciprocity and manifests completely the great dignity of human sexuality as a constitutive dimension of man's being as an image of God.

Given this outlook, one can perhaps understand the depth of what is said in number II, 4, which represents the cornerstone of the entire Instruction.

It is the fruit of a strongly unified conception of man, *corpore et anima unus* (*Gaudium et Spes*, no. 14). The anthropological perspective of man as a "unified totality," stated in *Familiaris Consortio*, finds, in the first part of Pope John Paul II's Catecheses on the *Theology of the Body*, a basic foundation that enables the Instruction to posit the first of two affirmations contained in this decisive paragraph: procreation is deprived of its proper perfection when it is not willed as the fruit of the conjugal act.

Based on this principle, read in the light of a correct theology of sexuality, it is easy to proceed to the second: the unity of the human being and the dignity of his origin demand that human procreation be the fruit of a specific conjugal act of love between spouses. In effect, this means that if, because of the *imago*, the fertility of human sexuality is linked, in a mysterious but not arbitrary fashion, to the very fruitfulness of the Trinitarian life, such that there corresponds to the Trinity—with a capital "T"—a small "t" trinity, despite there being a massive dissimilarity, then the *child*, the third subject of the triad, enjoys from the beginning the full dignity that is derived from his taking part in the *imago*. Indeed, from the union of man and woman another human is born, *this human*, who must therefore be respected from his conception as a person (cf. I, 1). He is not a mere instance of the human species, as he would be if human sexuality was wholly identical to that of animals, and if man's body, including his most elementary instinctual biological dynamisms and the most hidden urges of his natural affectivity, were not permeated by God's creative intentionality. "I have produced a male child with the help of the LORD" (Gn 4:1), Eve says after having given birth to Cain. In this phrase is encapsulated the very mystery of nascent life, which essentially implies the specific act of conjugal love that is by its nature open to procreation. In this way do the spouses cooperate with God's creative action (cf. II, 4).

4. Do those men of today who are involved in the adventure of biomedical technology, which is a stupendous expression of obedience to the divine command to *subdue the cosmos*, know how to make room for *Donum Vitae*'s appeal? In order to do so they will have to bow down to consider the integral meaning of man as a creature made in God's image, thus recognizing the fallacy of the so-called *technological imperative*. Even in this they will be aided by the prophetic appeal of the Church, who calls for an elementary consideration: no science and no technology are morally neutral (cf. Introduction, 2). They are all always dependent on an anthropology, that is, on a vision of man, from which specific ethical imperatives follow. Not everything that is technically possible is morally acceptable, since every medical act is not to be viewed only in its technical dimension; rather, it always has a relation to the integral good of the person (cf. II, 7).

In order to respect man in his integrity it is necessary to listen to the law that is not written but imprinted in our hearts. Its decrees arise from the very mystery of man created and redeemed.

If on account of love God humbled himself to create man from nothing and, still on account of love, in his Son Jesus Christ emptied himself to the point of death in order to redeem man by the Cross, why ought not man, when on account of love he wishes to generate, humble himself to listen to the law imprinted into the transcendent nature of his very body? *For our nature speaks to us, since insofar as we all have been made, we all come from a decision of Trinitarian love!* This is a substantial principle, without the acceptance of which man will never be able to understand affection, love, and sexuality. The importance of such a principle did not escape the great teachers of antiquity, or those of the Medieval Christians. It was not because they did not yet know the empirical-Galilean science, but because they possessed that Wisdom that we, too often, show ourselves unable to appreciate.

Respect for Human Embryos

DIONIGI TETTAMANZI
Instructor of Moral and Pastoral Theology
at the Seminary of Milan

The recent document from the Congregation for the Doctrine of the Faith is organized in three parts, the first of which is dedicated to "Respect for Human Embryos." The argument unfolds according to the literary genre of "question and answer": these latter are formulated at the beginning in a summary fashion and are then reiterated with a fuller, more developed argument.

The Gift of Life

What is said in the "Introduction" about the reality of human life is essential for a full grasp of this first section. The very first lines establish the "fundamental principle" that must lie "at the center of one's reflection": "The gift of life that God the Creator and Father has entrusted to man calls him to appreciate the inestimable value of what he has been given and to take responsibility for it."

Now the inestimable value of human life emerges from the Church's doctrine on man. The document outlines a synthesis of the key elements, starting with the principle of *absolute respect* for the life of every human being from the moment of conception. This principle is justified by a series of reasons that are mutually coordinated: man is the only creature on earth whom God has "willed for itself" (*Gaudium et Spes*, no. 24); the spiritual soul of every man is "immediately created" by God; the splendor of the Creator's image shines on man's entire being. Thus are posited the bases for life's *sacredness*: it is sacred because, from the beginning, it carries "the creative action of God" and because it remains forever in a special relation with God, its sole end. The sacredness of life is also based on and demanded by *God's exclusive and unique lordship* over it: "God alone is the Lord of life, from its beginning to its end." From this it follows that "no one can, in any circumstance, claim for himself the right to destroy directly an innocent human being." Whoever dares usurp the divine lordship over life has objectively placed himself in a position amounting to sacrilege.

Corresponding to the absolute respect for human life is the *inviolability* of the right to life of every innocent human being. But what is the root, and at the same time, the force, of such inviolability? It is the human *person* as such: it is his incomparable value as God's image that makes him inviolable in the gift of life that the Creator has bestowed upon him. The person's inviolability is revealed and asserted in the inviolability of human life.

Here we come to the decisive and driving question: Is even the human embryo, from the beginning of his existence, a human person, such that he is inviolable in his right to life and demands an absolute and unconditional respect?

This is the first question addressed by the Instruction: "What respect is due to the human embryo, taking into account his nature and identity?"

We have described this question as "decisive," decisive in the literal sense of the word, since its answer will decide, that is justify and necessitate, the moral solution to different problems that have arisen from the artificial interventions on the human embryo. It is at the same time the "driving" question, if we are to proceed not by following "prejudice," but rather "rationality." To invoke, as some do, the "right" to experiment on human embryo-fetuses for the benefit of scientific development, or to do research aimed at a possible cure for illnesses that have so far been incurable, as well as to insist on legislative projects for the use of human embryo-fetuses, without having previously defined, with necessary seriousness, the proper identity, or as they say, the "state" or "status" of the human embryo, signifies a radical contradiction of an elementary and irrefutable requirement of rationality toward itself, and, therefore, a requirement of justice with respect to the embryo. One cannot abandon oneself to the "opinions" of few or many, which are, most of the time, subject to socio-cultural pressure from widely varying groups, when what is at stake is not one "opinion" among many "opinions," but the "reality" of human life, that is the "human being" himself in the inviolability of his personal dignity and his right to life.

The Nature and Identity of the Human Embryo

For her part, the Church reasserts her "constant and certain" doctrine, repeated again to contemporary man by Vatican II: "From the moment of its conception life must be guarded with the greatest care, while abortion and infanticide are unspeakable crimes" (*Gaudium et Spes*, no. 51). Echoing the conciliar affirmation, the recent *Charter on the Rights of the Family* writes, "Human life must be respected and protected absolutely from the moment of conception" (article 4).

It must now be asked, what is the meaning and import of this doctrine when confronted with "the current debates concerning the beginning of human life, concerning the individuality of the human being and concerning the identity of the human person"? The document reconsiders and reiterates what the same Congregation wrote in the *Declaration on Procured Abortion* in 1974. Leaving aside the completely subjective and "theoretical" debate regarding the moment of rational animation, the Declaration vigorously reaffirmed the "practical" position, which entailed a grave moral obligation to follow the road of certainty: "From a moral point of view this is certain: even if a doubt existed concerning whether the fruit of conception is already a human person, it is objectively a grave sin to dare to risk murder. 'The one who will be a man is already one' (Tertullian, *Apologeticum*, IX, 8: *PL* I, 371-372)" (no. 13).

Let us now read from the Instruction: "The Magisterium has not expressly committed itself to an affirmation of a philosophical nature." At the same time, on the practical level, the Instruction on the one hand states, in explicit terms, that "the human being is to be respected and treated as a person from the moment of conception; and therefore from that same moment his rights as a person must be recognized"; on the other hand, it seems to encourage a more basic anthropological reflection. To stimulate such reflection, we now have the very "conclusions of science regarding the human embryo." Science cannot go beyond its own specific competence: "Certainly no experimental datum can be in itself sufficient to bring us to the recognition of a spiritual soul"; but (philosophical-theological) reason cannot fail to ask itself, "How could a human individual not be a human person?" This consideration and its answer are subject to rational inquiry. But it seems to us that it is not without a particular significance that the document should have posed the question in an explicit manner.

The Embryo Like Every Other Human Person

From all this there emerges the *fundamental criterion* for responding to the different problems arising from artificial interventions on human embryos: since the embryo must be treated as a person: (1) he must be recognized as possessing the *same rights as "every other human being"*: hence the categorical "no" to every possible "discrimination," insofar as such would constitute the direct negation of the "equality" of all human beings, an equality based on the unique, identical, and universal worth of human beings (their personal dignity); (2) he must be *defended* in his integrity and his life, just as he must be *cared for* (and healed, to the extent that it is possible), in the same way as every other human being.

It is obvious that, in the application of such precepts, one cannot fail to take into account the specific situation of the human embryo-fetus: one must consider, for example, the free and informed consent of the parents or of the mother, which would be required for the carrying out of some intervention on the human embryo-fetus; one must consider the delicate and arduous application of the risk-benefit principle of proportionality, given the particular risk of interventions at the very early phases, which, at least at present, have very little therapeutic potential; one must consider too—and differently than one considers adult cases—the unique therapeutic goal, that is, what is the good of the embryo-fetus himself, which will legitimize the intervention done on a human being who is incapable of consent.

Different Interventions

In the application of the fundamental criterion, the document follows a logical order, addressing firstly the problem of prenatal diagnosis, which allows one to know the conditions of the embryo-fetus in the maternal uterus; and then the problem of operational interventions, which are distinguished based on their intended goals: the goal might be therapeutic (cure and healing) or scientific (research and experimentation).

As with every other human being, *therapeutic intervention* for the benefit of the human embryo-fetus is morally legitimate if it is truly "therapeutic," that is, if it is geared "toward its healing, the improvement of its condition of health, or its individual survival," if it respects the integrity and life of the human embryo-fetus, and if it does not carry disproportionate risks.

The problem of *research* and *experimentation* is more complex. After having accurately specified the terms of "research" and "experimentation," which are often used in an equivocal and ambiguous manner, the document (1) *rejects medical research* on living embryos "unless there is a moral certainty of not causing harm to the life or integrity of the unborn child and the mother, and on condition that the parents have given their free and informed consent to the procedure" to be performed on the embryo; here we are dealing with "research," that is with "any inductive-deductive process which aims at promoting the systematic observation of a given phenomenon in the human field or at verifying a hypothesis arising from previous observations"; (2) with respect to *experimentation, the document distinguishes between still-living and dead embryos*.

In the first case "*experimentation on embryos which is not directly therapeutic is illicit*." From everything discussed thus far, the reason for this illegitimacy is obvious: "To use human embryos or fetuses as the object or instrument of experimentation constitutes a crime against their dignity as human beings having a right to the same respect that is due to the child already born and to every human person."

The second case involves the respect for the corpses of human embryos or fetuses, "just like the remains of other human beings." Potential interventions are legitimate on the same conditions, namely the certainty of death, the consent of the parents or of the mother, the exclusion of any complicity in procured abortion, the absence of the danger of scandal, and the rejection of any commercial practice.

In vitro fertilization has opened up another situation: *the production of human embryos precisely for the sake of research* and experimentation. The moral solution to this problem comes from the principle that "human embryos obtained *in vitro* are human beings and subjects with rights: their dignity and right to life must be respected from the first moment of their existence." It follows then that it is immoral to (1) *produce* embryos destined to be harvested as disposable "biological material"; (2) voluntarily *distribute* them; (3) *expose* them either to grave and disproportionate risks or even to death. Once these embryos have been produced *in vitro*, they are exposed to an "absurd fate": a morally acceptable outcome for those embryos not transferred to the body of the mother is impossible, which signals unequivocally the moral impracticability of the *in vitro* fertilization procedure.

The final problem comes from additional forms of *biological or genetic manipulation* on human embryos. The document mentions the cross-fertilization of human and animal gametes, the gestation of human embryos in the uteruses of animals, the hypothesis or project of an artificial uterus, the obtaining of a human being without any connection to sexuality ("twin fission," cloning, parthenogenesis), the freezing of embryos, the selection of sex and of other predetermined qualities. Now all these forms of manipulation are contrary to the personal dignity of the embryo, and every one of them is contrary to it relative to the particular values and requirements of such dignity, including integrity and life, conception within marriage, maternal gestation, the uniqueness and unrepeatability of the person, his identity, and his belonging to the human, not the animal, world.

You Did It to Me

Let us conclude by highlighting the outlook chosen by the document: it begins with the human embryo-fetus, proclaiming his personal dignity and the rights that follow therefrom, and demanding that he be absolutely respected.

The dominant social-cultural outlook, to which various scientists, politicians and legislators, couples and doctors, end up submitting, is different: it begins with the adult world, with their presumed "rights" (which are really their "desires"). This brings with it a danger, one which is far too evident: the danger of failing to attend to, or even of failing to recognize the rights of the little ones, in this case of the human embryo-fetuses.

It is worthwhile to consider that the very consistency of democracy is at stake. As was observed, universality and equality are the principles that support and allow for the growth of democracy: *all men are equal in their dignity!* As history documents, the democratic journey has been long and wearying, and still is. But there is no doubt that its development is inseparably linked to the demolition of all the barriers that have divided and continue to divide the different "groups" of men, pitting them against one another and urging them on to ever-varying forms of discrimination and injustice. *Today a "new" category looks out on the history of humanity*, asking to take their rightful place in democracy: it is the group of these little ones, these smallest human beings who are the embryo-fetuses. The challenge has been offered to the adults, on whom alone depends the real recognition of the equal human dignity of the embryo-fetuses.

In this sense "beginning with the last" and ending with those who make themselves "first" is a profoundly human requirement. Above all it is an evangelical requirement, and whoever listens to the words of Christ, "Whatever you did for one of these least brothers of mine, you did for me" (Mt 25:40), can understand the radicality it entails. It is precisely with these most luminous and disturbing words that the Instruction ends, pointing out that they yield today "a new and particular echo." The reference is clear: it is to human embryos. These are the least among "Christ's" brethren. The Church, as faithful spouse of the Lord Jesus, takes their part: for it is there that she finds her Spouse, the Son of Man.

The Dignity of Human Procreation

ALBERT CHAPELLE
Instructor of Moral Theology at the Brussels Institute for Theological Studies

The second part of the Instruction *Donum Vitae* deals with various interventions on human procreation, and more precisely with "the different technical procedures directed toward obtaining a human conception in a manner other than the sexual union of man and woman" (II, Introduction); the Instruction speaks of IVF and ET (*in vitro* fertilization and embryonic transfer) and of artificial insemination.

It is well to carefully examine the structure of this second part. A preliminary point situates the forms of artificial procreation within the culture that has rendered them possible. The expository plan of the document distinguishes between heterologous artificial fertilization ("techniques used to obtain a human conception artificially by the use of gametes coming from at least one donor other than the spouses who are joined in marriage") and homologous artificial fertilization (which uses "the gametes of the two spouses joined in marriage" II, 4-6); the moral consideration of these forms of artificial procreation thus appears tied to the matrimonial institution. After the moral evaluation of these procedures, the document considers issues having to do with the conscience of the doctors (II, 7) and to that of sterile couples (II, 8).

The perspective from which the techniques of artificial fertilization are approached is a realistic one. "Development of the practice of *in vitro* fertilization has required innumerable fertilizations and destructions of human embryos" (II, Introduction). "The connection between *in vitro* fertilization and the voluntary destruction of human embryos" reveals a logic of violence and domination, which is sometimes not even noticed by the very ones who adhere to it. The facts of the matter and the logic of a research that claims to deal out life and death on command are constitutive of the abortive "mentality" and abortive practices, without which, according to the agents' own views, IVF and ET could not have been realized.

The Moral Dimension of Science and Technology

This page should be read in the light of the Introduction, which calls for science and technology to be at the service of the human person (Introduction, 2). The evocation of a civilization that would aspire to dominion over life, at the price of the death of human beings, is illuminated by the allusion to different attempts at arbitrary intervention on the chromosomal or genetic heritage; selectivity (I, 5); eugenics (II, Introduction); and euthanasia (cf. I, 4, no. 31) are among the consequences of this promethean project, whose atheistic inspiration is undeniable.

Artificial modes of procreation entail decisive choices for civilization. Nonetheless, the examination of their intrinsic and objective moral quality cannot be carried out merely by evoking these grave "circumstances" and consequences, not to say murders. These "abuses do not exempt one from a further and thorough ethical study of the techniques of artificial procreation considered in themselves" (II, Introduction). The cultural context is nonetheless helpful in identifying the real dimensions of the moral question that has been posed to humanity since the discovery of newly acquired powers over man's biological existence.

This specification of outlook introduces a precise examination of the intrinsic morality of the procedures in question. The plan of the Instruction distinguishes between heterologous and homologous fertilization. "Every human being is always to be accepted as a gift and blessing of God. However, from the moral point of view a truly responsible procreation vis-à-vis the unborn child must be the fruit of marriage" (II, 1). Before making any other clarification, this teaching requires the distinction between the moral specificity of the forms of artificial procreation, regarding the extent to which they operate in greater or lesser conformity with and respect for the propriety of marriage.

Heterologous Artificial Fertilization

The moral problem with this procedure comes from the separation it entails between "genetic" parenthood, "gestational" parenthood, and "educational" responsibility (II, 2).

The Instruction responds with two points:

1) It reviews the question: Why should "marriage and . . . its indissoluble unity" be considered "the only setting worthy of truly responsible procreation" (II, 1)? The Instruction recalls the classic answer and its four principal

arguments: the unity of matrimony and the good of the child, of the parents, and of civil society. At the same time, it clarifies the traditional doctrine, "The fidelity of the spouses in the unity of marriage involves reciprocal respect of their right to become a father and a mother only through each other."

2) Thus are brought together the elements that allow for the evaluation as to whether heterologous fertilization can be in moral conformity with the dignity of the spouses and the truth of marriage. The document reasserts the Church's very ancient doctrine, applying it in all its rigor. Just as every sexual union outside of marriage is contrary to the fidelity of the spouses, in the same way, the spouses have the exclusive, objective, and inalienable right of not procreating unless it is through each other. The child, moreover, has the right not only of being conceived and brought into the world in marriage, but also by marriage and through marriage, through the acts of the parents. Finally, every deliberate disassociation of the different parental functions is contrary to the vocation of spouses called to a paternity and a maternity that integrates the physical, psychical, moral, and spiritual dimensions of their being.

These lines of thought and their implications at the social level entail a negative judgment on any kind of heterologous artificial fertilization. The document specifies (in case there should be any doubt) that so-called "surrogate" motherhood is morally illicit for the same reasons (II, 3).

Homologous Artificial Insemination

Artificial homologous fertilization poses another type of problem, in that here we are dealing with IVF and ET or with artificial insemination between the spouses.

Here the Instruction proceeds in the same way as it did with respect to forms of homologous artificial fertilization: it recalls the traditional principles (II, 4), and then applies them to the techniques under investigation: IVF and ET (II, 5) and artificial insemination (II, 6). The "propriety" of marriage is not sufficient for clarifying the moral legitimacy of the different modes of homologous artificial fertilization; it is true that these latter procedures, in contrast to forms of heterologous artificial fertilization, do not challenge the unity and indissolubility of marriage. Instead the consideration focuses on the doctrine of the "goods" of marriage, and of the meanings of the conjugal act: what bond is required from the moral perspective—not just the bond between procreation and matrimony (II, 1)—but more specifically the bond between procreation and the conjugal act (II, 4)? The response to this question will strictly determine the moral evaluation of the "technique used to (artificially) obtain a human conception using the gametes of the two spouses joined in marriage" (II, Introduction).

The bond that is required between procreation and the "conjugal act which is suitable in itself for the procreation of offspring, to which marriage is ordered by its nature and by which the spouses become one flesh" (*Code of Canon Law*, c. 10, cited in II, 4b) is established through a reflection laid out in three points.

The Nature of Marriage

The first point (a) argues from the intimate connection between the goods and between the meanings of marriage; the second (b) and the third (c) points support and expand the first argument by means of a consideration of the personal character of the union between the spouses (b) and the procreation of the child (c).

a) The first argument (II, 4a) takes as its point of departure "the inseparable connection, established by God, which man on his own initiative may not break, between the unitive significance and the procreative significance which are both inherent to the marriage act" (*Humanae Vitae*, no. 12). This principle, which is founded on the nature of marriage and on the intimate connection between its goods, carries well-known implications at the level of responsible fatherhood and motherhood; it also illuminates the moral problem regarding homologous artificial fertilization.

The Instruction combines the traditional doctrine on the goods of marriage with the teaching of *Humanae Vitae* and of *Gaudium et Spes* on the meanings and values of the conjugal act. Due to this integration, called for by Pope John Paul II (II, 4, n43), the Instruction posits an "analogy" between contraception and homologous artificial fertilization: "Contraception deliberately deprives the conjugal act of its openness to procreation and in this way brings about a voluntary dissociation of the ends of marriage. Homologous artificial fertilization, in seeking a procreation which is not the fruit of a specific act of conjugal union, objectively effects an analogous separation between the goods and the meanings of marriage."

This way of thinking, already suggested by Pope Pius XII (n40), vividly highlights the moral object and the voluntary character ("deliberately deprives"—"brings about a voluntary dissociation"—"seeking a procreation"—"objectively effects an analogous separation"): abstracting from the circumstances or the intentions, it is the *volitum*, the object willed, that determines the act of the will at a moral level. Only what is morally willed can be morally wicked: "But *from the moral point of view* [that is, from the point of view of the act of the will] procreation is deprived of its proper perfection when it is not *desired* as the fruit of the conjugal act, that is to say of the specific act of the spouses' union."

This first argument appears, after the manner of *Humanae Vitae*, to be a logical consequence of the doctrine regarding "the goods of marriage" and "the meanings of the conjugal act." But the doctrine is again taken up and expressed here in terms belonging to an anthropology and a metaphysics inspired by the catecheses of Pope John Paul II (cited in footnote 43).

b) The bond between the goods of marriage finds its origin and basis in the unity of the human being, "*corpore et anima unus*" (*Gaudium et Spes*, no. 14, 1, cited in the Introduction, 3). This doctrine of the person—body and spiritual soul—yields a deeper understanding of the teaching regarding the goods of marriage, and that in two directions.

1. The language of finality is almost never used, even if it reappears in terms of "values" (II, 4). The distinctions between *finis operis* and *finis operantis*, the secondary end and the primary end, do not surface. One will not again encounter even the distinction between *opus personarum* and *opus naturae*, which was too often reduced to the distinction between the moral and affective level on the one hand, and between the physiological and social level on the other. Goods remain as desirable (appetable) "values," but they are affirmed in the terminology of the person's *finis cui*, of the dignity of his being and of the generosity (*diffusivum sui*) of his particular acts.

2. The doctrine of the human person (of the human being) and of his act is made explicit in the logic of generosity and gift that belongs to love. Consequently, the intimate connection between the goods of marriage (union and procreation) is contained within the "language of the body" as the expression and pledge of the persons' union.

This good is expressed chiefly "on the part of the spouses" (b): "The conjugal act by which the couple mutually expresses their self-gift at the same time expresses openness to the gift of life. . . . In order to respect the language of their bodies and their natural generosity, the conjugal union must take place with respect for its openness to procreation; and the procreation of a person must be the fruit and the result of married love."

c) The same logic of generosity and love allows for a deeper awareness of the dignity of human procreation "on the part of the person of the child": "In his . . . origin, the child must be respected and recognized as equal in personal dignity to those who give him life. The human person must be accepted in his parents' act of union and love . . . ," and it is in this way that he will be associated with communion. "The generation of a child must therefore be the fruit of that mutual giving which is realized in the conjugal act wherein the spouses cooperate . . . in the work of the Creator who is Love."

The "origin of a person" must be the result of a gift. The generation of the child should not here be expressed in terms of reproducing the human species, but from the perspective of a procreation arising from the love of persons and destined to be in communion with them.

This anthropological restatement of the doctrine of the goods of marriage leads to the recognition, within the union of the spouses and in the generation of the child to be born, of those acts proper to the original dignity of human persons. The goods of marriage cannot be dissociated without contradicting this logic of generation and love; the latter recognizes the person in his origin and recognizes him as a gift.

This personalistic mediation adds nothing to the traditional moral doctrine but rather supports its moral obligations and shows its significance. It enables us to understand the union of spouses and human procreation, not on the model of animal sexuality and reproduction, but from the standpoint of the mystery of generation and love, where the person is originated and where the gift of oneself is realized. The Instruction does not invoke the possible Trinitarian foundations for this "personology," but it does soberly reach the following logical conclusion: "The procreation of a human person" must "be brought about [that is, willed] as the fruit of the conjugal act specific to the love between spouses."

The discussion on the morality of homologous artificial fertilization depends on these anthropological and moral principles. Nonetheless, these are nothing if not a reiteration of the "traditional doctrine relating to the goods of marriage" reflected in the light of the dignity of the person (II, 4). This is why the document may expressly refer to the positions of the Magisterium (II, 4) in pronouncing against the moral legitimacy of homologous *in vitro* fertilization (II, 5).

With this goal the Instruction proceeds in four successive steps. It manifests "the very nature of homologous IVF and ET," considered abstractly from the intentions (for example, as a remedy for sterility) and the moral circumstances. "The process of IVF and ET must be judged in itself and cannot borrow its definitive moral quality from the totality of conjugal life of which it becomes part nor from the conjugal acts which may precede or follow it." This has to do with the moral doctrine of distinguishing the object from the circumstances or the intention. It was also reasserted in *Humanae Vitae*, number 14, with regard to contraception (II, n48).

"The very nature of homologous IVF and ET" must therefore be analyzed "abstracting from the link with procured abortion."

The Instruction characterizes IVF and ET by describing it with the following elements of the *human act* that are involved: the dissociation of the conjugal act and the technical actions that oversee the fertilization; the realization "outside the bodies of the couple through actions of third parties whose competence and technical activity determine the success of the procedure"; the establishment of a domination by technology over the origin, identity, and destiny of the human person.

Cooperators with God for the Gift of Life

3. This characterization highlights the *moral specificity* of homologous IVF and ET. *In vitro* fertilization comes from a technological action that oversees the fertilization; it is therefore "neither in fact achieved nor positively willed as the expression and fruit of a specific act of the conjugal union" (II, 5). Therefore—and this is the conclusion that derives from the absence of the morally required link between procreation and the conjugal act (II, 4)—in homologous IVF and ET, *the generation of the human person is objectively deprived of its proper perfection: namely, that of being the result and fruit of a conjugal act* in which the spouses can become 'cooperators with God for giving life to a new person.'" This citation from *Familiaris Consortio*, number 14, illustrates the theological relevance of the argument, which is approached in terms of generation, person, and gift.

4. Once the moral specificity of homologous IVF and ET has been determined, it still remains to render explicit *the moral judgment given by the Church*. This is formulated in two ways:

a) The "simple case" has been studied by moralists in order to describe homologous IVF and ET in its moral objectivity—abstracting from the subjective intentions and the morally aggravating circumstances ("compromise with the abortive practice of destroying embryos and with masturbation"). This is characterized as "a technique which is morally illicit," insofar as it deprives human procreation of the dignity that is proper and connatural to it.

b) Homologous IVF and ET is not "marked by all that ethical negativity"—by the specific malice—that one finds in extra-conjugal procreation. Nonetheless, "in conformity with the traditional doctrine relating to the goods of marriage and the dignity of the person," the Church states, with the voice of her Magisterium, that she remains "opposed from the moral point of view to homologous *in vitro* fertilization. Such fertilization is in itself illicit and in opposition to the dignity of procreation," from which the person should originate; it also opposes the dignity of "the conjugal union," where the reciprocal giving of the spouses and the gift of life to a new human person should take place.

The Bond Between the Conjugal Act and Procreation

The moral value of the bond between procreation and the conjugal union, and the illegitimacy of homologous *in vitro* fertilization are closely linked in the doctrine of the present document.

The content of *Donum Vitae* corresponds to that of *Humanae Vitae*: its line of reasoning is near to that of *Familiaris Consortio*; its inspiration resembles that of *Gaudium et Spes*; its doctrinal development finds sustenance even in the teachings of Popes Leo XII, Pius XI, and Pius XII. In keeping with these different magisterial authorities, the Congregation for the Doctrine of the Faith today illuminates the internal coherence and relevance of a common doctrine.

Even the "teaching of the Magisterium" concerning homologous artificial insemination is taken up and reasserted from the same perspective. "If the technical means facilitates the conjugal act or helps it to reach its natural objectives, it can be morally acceptable. If, on the other hand, the procedure were to replace the conjugal act, it is morally illicit" (II, 6). This moral precision "is based on the Church's doctrine concerning the connection between the conjugal union and procreation and on a consideration of the personal nature of the conjugal act and of human procreation." The same explicit consideration in *Gaudium et Spes* (no. 51, 3)—which is cited here—invites us to see "masturbation, through which the sperm is normally obtained" for artificial fertilization, as an act that "remains deprived of its unitive meaning" of the "sexual relationship called for by the moral order."

The teaching on the illegitimacy of artificial modes of homologous and heterologous fertilization is doubtless more precise than anyone might have supposed. At the end of the Instruction, the Congregation for the Doctrine of the Faith addresses an appeal and an encouragement to theologians and moralists, "that they study more deeply and make even more accessible to the faithful the contents of the teaching of the Church's Magisterium" (Conclusion, p. 39). Undoubtedly we will have to reflect more deeply on the personal dignity of the human embryo, of conjugal union and of procreation. The uniqueness that the person reveals in his origin, and the fullness that he manifests in the gift of himself, has not ceased to illuminate the mystery of life and love among men.

The Exemplary Observance of a "Moral Norm"

Before concluding, the Instruction of the Congregation for the Doctrine of Faith examines two cases of conscience, resolving them in the light of the doctrine that has been proposed.

1. The first case deals with the intervention by the doctor and by the medical professional on human procreation. We recall the principle: medical treatment, ordered to the integral good of the person, must respect the specifically human values of sexuality.

From this it follows that it is good to aid the conjugal act, but from the moral perspective the medical intervention must not replace "the conjugal act in order to obtain a procreation which is neither its result nor its fruit."

A threefold appeal is formulated in order to request the practical respect of these norms: it is directed to doctors, to Catholic researchers, to "the medical and nursing staff of Catholic hospitals and clinics . . . who are often Religious." It does not constitute the promulgation of a positive ecclesiastical law, but a request for the exemplary observance of a "moral norm," which is in itself universally valid.

2. A final situation attracts the attention of the Vatican Instruction: the suffering of conjugal sterility. This suffering is to be recognized and respected as a "sharing in a particular way in the Lord's Cross, the source of spiritual fruitfulness." Nonetheless, nothing confers on the spouses a true and proper right to a child; a child is a gift, not something owed. On the contrary, it is the child who has "the right . . . to be the fruit of the specific act of the conjugal love of his parents" (cf. II, 5), "and he also has the right to be respected as a person from the moment of his conception" (cf. I, 1). These two fundamental principles of the Instruction illuminate the outlook of morally valid research in the struggle against sterility.

This appeal allows us to see even in the person of the child a living pledge and criterion of the beauty and dignity of the beginnings of human life.

Aspects of Medical Deontology

ELIO SGRECCIA
Director of the Bioethics Center of the Catholic University of Rome

Today the image of the doctor is subject to various and conflicting impressions. On the one hand, legislative ordinances in many governments have organized health care as a service of the state with respect to the citizens, accentuating its centralized management, and this situation may, along with evident advantages, also lead to the risk of reducing the doctor to the status of a functionary of health care, contractually dependent on the health care organization. The contract or agreement with the patient risks becoming secondary and fragile when compared to the contract with the state.

On the other hand, the demand for health that society promotes is no longer limited to the classic realm of medicine, prevention, cure, and rehabilitation, according to a personalistic concept of health and according to the therapeutic principle that has always been the doctor's deontological guide. Health is often understood as being "full" well-being, and therefore, a fuller demand is established that goes beyond the limits of therapeutic medicine and becomes described as "the medicine of the desires." The desire for a child at all costs may be located within this new demand.

There is another reason technology in the biomedical field has been willing to move outside the classic and traditional meaning of the medical act: technology as applied to medicine, while it better allows for the healing of illness, also provides instruments for the manipulation of human life.

In this situation of competing forces, we must enumerate a final, grave threat to the medical profession: the loss or obfuscation of its ethical-deontological status, which has always been based on the relationship or agreement between doctor and patient, understood as an interpersonal and trusting alliance, founded on intangible and transcendent values: the respect for the person and for the life of every human being.

Through their organizations and according to their best traditions, doctors have been struggling laudably to keep their own ethical and deontological identity safe from the temptations of bureaucratization and free from the demand for interventions that may be purely technological or simply instrumental in the service of simple hedonistic or ideologically diversified desires.

The Instruction of the Congregation for the Doctrine of the Faith constitutes, under this heading, an aid and a clarification in confirming what is the role of the doctor with regard to the person and in particular with regard to issues of procreation.

The document, underscoring the sacredness and intangibility of human life from its emergence, and the personalistic and nontransferable character of the procreative act, situates the worth of the person and inalienability of his values at the very height of the medical act and at the very center of medical activity; and thus, with this orientation, it reinforces the autonomy and the identity of the medical role. The ethical-deontological identity and the defense of life and of the human person stand or fall together, like mirror images.

We can test this reflection by analyzing the most significant passages of the document.

The Doctor with Respect to Nascent Human Life

"The human being must be respected—as a person—from the very first instant of his existence" (Instruction, I, 1).

The newly conceived individual comes under consideration, as he should in the logic of ethical-anthropological reason, in three points that determine his value: firstly, from the point of view of the Creator; secondly, from the point of view of the dignity of marriage and of the procreative act; and finally, in terms of its effect, the human person, who originates at conception.

With respect to this value, in virtue of which embryonic life takes on the ethical character of a person, the doctor's attitude should be one of respect, of therapeutic support, and of defense. Regarding the interventions on the embryo, the document affirms, "One must uphold as licit procedures carried out on the human embryo which respect the life and integrity of the embryo and do not involve disproportionate risks for it but are directed toward its healing, the improvement of its condition of health, or its individual survival" (Instruction, I, 3).

It is the *therapeutic principle* that is reaffirmed, along with what the document states about the obligation of obtaining the parents' consent for every intervention on the embryo and on the fetus, even during a point of therapy, in conformity with the principles that medical deontology itself posits when confronting interventions on minors.

Regarding the procedure of *prenatal diagnosis*, which today is very often used with the goal of controlling and selecting preborn children, the Instruction positively underscores the validity/legitimacy of the exploratory-diagnostic procedure, which is in itself independent of the possible uses to which it is put; all the same, it reiterates the condemnation of the abortive intention and of any use directed to the elimination of fetuses affected with malformations or hereditary diseases. In other words, the behavior of the couple and the doctor must be the same as it would in the case of diagnoses made on behalf of a child or even an adult who suffers from some handicap.

"If prenatal diagnosis respects the life and integrity of the embryo and the human fetus and is directed toward its safeguarding or healing, then the procedure is said to be a positive one" (Instruction, I, 2).

In prenatal diagnosis, therefore, as regards the techniques, which at this point carry excessive risks, and given the current mindset, which promotes the direct suppression of defective fetuses, the expert administering the diagnosis (doctor or geneticist) must be committed to a correct procedure and an honest and discreet dialogue that demands a combination of the duty to respect the truth and the duty to respect life, as well as the attendant commitment of responsibility and solidarity.

One cannot ignore the document's tone of openness to more advanced informative scientific procedures, which allow for a knowledge of the human being even before his birth, nor the ethical clarity in defending against any perverse utilization of them. The one who mediates this balance is once again the expert or professional who gives the diagnosis, to whom are entrusted the life of the unborn child and the concern of the couple.

Just as a balance has been approved regarding the competence of the scientist and the researcher, so too with the teaching on research and experimentation. While the research in itself has not been condemned when it is observational and also free of risk, there is a reassertion of the superiority of the worth of the unborn child's life, both as compared to the usefulness of science and as compared to utilitarian, socio-economic pressures. The Declaration of Helsinki (the ethical principles of the World Medical Association), issued in 1964, affirms the same principle for human research in its general outlines. The prerequisite conditions for research on persons, whether minors or adults, extend also to the need for consent.

Nevertheless, the document introduces a very delicate distinction between research and experimentation: the first may proceed via study and observation, and can leave unharmed the human being in question; the second has the goal of testing out technical procedures or pharmaceuticals, and uses the human being as an instrument or test subject. The latter is not to be performed on the embryo, since he cannot give his consent, nor can the consent of related representatives substitute for his, due to the inevitable risks of experimentation on the embryo.

"Medical research must refrain from operations on live embryos, unless there is a moral certainty of not causing harm to the life or integrity of the unborn child and the mother, and on condition that the parents have given their free and informed consent to the procedure" (Instruction, I, 4).

"If the embryos are living, whether viable or not, they must be respected just like any other human person; experimentation on embryos which is not directly therapeutic is illicit . . . Moreover, experimentation on embryos and fetuses always involves risk, and indeed in most cases it involves the certain expectation of harm to their physical integrity or even their death."

The image and the role of the doctor is consequently recognized even in his character as researcher, as included within the service to the truth and to the life of the individual human, which is the emblem of his dignity and the ethical boundary of his conduct.

The condemnation of the experimental procedures that have been unleashed against the embryos, the creation of embryos for experimental reasons, and the genetic manipulation of embryos (Instruction, I, 5 and 6) at the same time constitute the rejection of the image of the doctor as enslaved to social utilitarianism or to the technocratic establishment.

The Doctor and Procreation

The courageous claim made by the Instruction regarding the procreative act, which is identified as belonging exclusively to the expression of spousal and parental love, and the consequent condemnation of every reduction of procreation to an act of biological-technological production, and finally the rejection of every procedure on the part of the gynecology doctor that replaces the very act of procreation, all restore to the doctor the function of helping and supporting procreation; in other words, they recognize his therapeutic mission, understood in its proper subsidiary significance.

"The humanization of medicine, which is insisted upon today by everyone, requires respect for the integral dignity of the human person first of all in the act and at the moment in which the spouses transmit life to a new person" (Instruction, II, 7).

It is within the sphere of the person and of procreation that God is present as Creator, and within which the spouses act as ministers of the gift of life. It is within this sphere that the limits of the doctor and of the gynecologist are circumscribed.

"Medicine which seeks to be ordered to the integral good of the person must respect the specifically human values of sexuality. The doctor is at the service of persons and of human procreation. He does not have the authority to dispose of them or to decide their fate" (Instruction, II, 7).

Doctors, however, like all scientists involved in the research of effective means of prevention and of valid therapies for sterility, are encouraged to be open to new ways of overcoming a difficulty, sterility, which painfully strikes many families.

"Scientists therefore are to be encouraged to continue their research with the aim of preventing the causes of sterility and of being able to remedy them so that sterile couples will be able to procreate in full respect for their own personal dignity and that of the child to be born" (Instruction, II, 8).

In the overcoming of the difficulties relative to the exercise of human sexuality and the work of supporting the procreative processes, the role of the doctor, both sexologist and gynecologist, is once more recognized in his work of therapist. He is therefore not deprived of his right and proper service to the integral good and the proper task of the spouses. Referencing the teaching of Pope Pius XII, the document sanctions the legitimacy of those procedures in which "the technical means is not a substitute for the conjugal act but serves to facilitate and to help so that the act attains its natural purpose" (Instruction, II, 6).

The Doctor in Society

The third part of the Instruction of the Congregation for the Doctrine of the Faith underscores the lamentable and well-known fact of the legalization of direct abortion, and it denounces the risk that the application of the techniques of artificial procreation will render this situation even more difficult in terms of the cultural, ideological, and political implications they bear.

Doctors, along with all men of good will, are exhorted to defend their right to "conscientious objection," in order that the laws facilitating and legitimizing direct abortion or the dissolution of the family be reformed. It also adds that "a movement of passive resistance to the legitimation of practices contrary to human life and dignity is beginning to make an ever sharper impression upon the moral conscience of many, especially among specialists in the biomedical sciences."

The medical profession is therefore called today to work toward not only the cure of disease and the defense of human life but also the cure of society in one of the gravest situations, namely that which comes from the inability to defend the life of everyone, and in particular the life of unborn children.

Doctors as individuals and within their associations, as well as Catholic institutions established for the defense and safeguarding of life and motherhood, have awaiting them, in the midst of a situation of ideological pressure and legislative dysfunction, a task for which the Church lends her support and her encouragement.

Morality and Civil Law

Gérard Mémeteau
Professor of Law
Vice-President of the Confédération des Juristes Catholiques

"It belongs to the Church always and everywhere to announce moral principles, even about the social order, and to render judgment concerning any human affairs insofar as the fundamental rights of the human person or the salvation of souls requires it" (*Code of Canon Law*, c. 747 §2).

The Congregation for the Doctrine of the Faith, with the Instruction of February 22, 1987, *On the Respect for Human Life in Its Origin and on the Dignity of Procreation*, has offered, in conformity with its mission, considerations of the utmost importance, not merely from the human point of view but also from that of the spiritual, concerning very delicate issues. Its teaching, which is formally and substantially in harmony with what it and the Supreme Pontiffs have developed on the problems of life and death, expresses the thought of the Magisterium of the Catholic Church. There is a distancing, however, from those bio-technical procedures that do not take into account the respect owed human life from its beginning, and owed the dignity of every person, regardless of his state of development and the quality of his life.

These behaviors "require the intervention of the political authorities and of the legislator, since an uncontrolled application of such techniques could lead to unforeseeable and damaging consequences for civil society." It is necessary to determine the normative function of the law with respect to scientific activities, so that these activities do not slip outside the legal sphere, establishing themselves as *faits accomplis*, to which the legislator and society are bound without previous discernment. And yet civil law cannot wholly protect someone who is treated as the property of another, nor therefore can civil law guarantee techniques that attack the most fundamental rights of someone who is "something more than nerves and tissue, blood and organs" (Pope Pius XII, Speech, January 30, 1945).

Hence the necessity of the public authority's intervention must align itself with the authority of natural limitations, that is, of the natural law.

I. The Necessity of Intervention by the Public Authority

While traditionally a doctor was reprimanded for not having recourse to all the techniques made available by the contemporary situation of science, now one begins to fear that these techniques will be applied in an overly far-reaching manner. Indeed, at this point there has been a transition from curative medicine to promethean medicine. "*Eritis sicut dei . . .*" "Various procedures now make it possible to intervene not only in order to assist but also to dominate the processes of procreation. . . . They might constitute progress in the service of man, but they also involve serious risks." No solution will be found to these grave difficulties without sufficient self-regulation.

A) The Seriousness of the Difficulty

1. The Appropriation of Life

Physical life safeguards the basis and the development of the other values of the person. Its inviolability is linked to that of the person, of which one cannot freely dispose. Certain juridical systems consecrate this value and its protection, declaring illicit any intervention on the human body without a therapeutic character.

The demands for interventions that are neither preventative nor curative, the severance of separate elements of the human body (except for necessary or benevolent cases), goes against the public order. Medical interventions that distance themselves from this finality, even if they are approved by the subject, automatically fall under penal law. The International Covenant on Civil and Political Rights (art. 7), the European Convention on Human Rights (art. 3), the American Convention on Human Rights (art. 5-2), and the African Charter on Human and Peoples' Rights (art. 5), prohibit cruel and degrading treatment. The Church's doctrine is not therefore absolutely isolated when it rejects every notion of making human life and the human body into property: "The natural moral law expresses and lays down the purposes, rights and duties which are based upon the bodily and spiritual nature of the human person."

Now there are two disturbing behaviors that should be noted. Certain legislations have made abortion legal under certain formal and specific conditions, and it is important to recall that, according to the law, without these conditions, the act remains subject to legal penalty. This phenomenon has led to the affirmation that abortion is the proper right of the woman, to the investigation of the doctor's negligence in the performance of this act, and finally to speculate about lawsuits for "wrongful life," filed by the child born handicapped, who would bring charges against his parents and the doctors for not having performed a eugenic abortion.

If abortion is the destruction of the embryo or the fetus in the womb, the Instruction notes that the practices of keeping human embryos alive *in vivo* or *in vitro* for experimental or commercial use and the destruction of the so-called "superfluous" embryos that are fertilized *in vitro* and not implanted—these practices are akin to abortion. These embryos are produced in order to "technically" facilitate the process of *in vitro* fertilization and embryonic transfer (IVF and ET), or for the sake of research, and their destruction is the destruction of human life: "It is therefore not in conformity with the moral law deliberately to expose to death human embryos obtained *in vitro* . . . Such deliberate destruction of human beings or their utilization for different purposes to the detriment of their integrity and life is contrary to the doctrine on procured abortion already recalled." Nor certainly is the act of freezing them any more moral, if one takes into account the risks involved. Nor is it appropriate to discuss how long the preservation lasts before the decision is made to destroy them.

It is a matter of principle not to attack created life (even artificially created life, although that's a different issue). The ethical presentation that accompanied the opinion of the (French) National Advisory Committee regarding "the research on human embryos *in vitro*" denounced the paradox of these risks of destroying life, brought about by the decision to create life, while maintaining all the while that the real concern was to find a solution to a lesser evil. The Instruction takes a firmer position, which it is able to do by not beginning from the starting point of a "happy medium." It would be inopportune, in penal law, to treat these behaviors as being equivalent to abortion. The principle of restrictive interpretation of criminal law would prevent it. However, one could speak of voluntary homicide.

The acts of scientific experimentation on the conceived baby, as opposed to those interventions that are therapeutic (this is the common distinction in deontology and in medical law), elicit the same reservations (cf. Pope John Paul II, Address, October 23, 1982). As far as prenatal diagnosis goes, its ambiguity (which has already been denounced when speaking about the cause or goal of the medical procedure used to diagnose) is ultimately underscored with respect to the abortion that may constitute its basis, and in light of which the diagnosis may be requested. Moreover, reference is made to the norm of proportionate reason, which, as has been noted, moral theology has borrowed from medical law, to ensure that the risks of this diagnosis are situated in relation to the foreseeable therapeutic advantages.

Even the dissociation of the process of fertilization is considered an act of domination over life, insofar as the individual makes himself "someone who gives life and death at will" (cf. the document "Vie et mort sur commande" of the Commission on the Family of the French Episcopate: *Doc. Cath.* 2 XII [1984], 1126). On this matter civil law poses some delicate questions about the maternal and paternal parenthood of the child born through methods of assisted procreation other than homologous artificial fertilization: questions about the legal presumptions of legitimate fatherhood, about motherhood, about the cases in which an investigation is opened regarding natural paternity, about adoption, about the act of disowning . . . all these articles will have to be rewritten! Is prenatal diagnosis perhaps entering into the arsenal of civil and penal evidence to be used in a legal setting? The Instruction did not need to respond to these problems: nonetheless it adds to this reflection the right of the child to be "conceived, carried in the womb, brought into the world, and brought up within marriage," and the duty of not achieving procreation except from within the combined biological and spiritual union of the parents. Nor may the baby be made "an object of scientific technology."

2. The Loss of the Human Dimension

In the end, it is this that is the principal problem, to know what is "human," and it therefore lies outside juridical processes, outside any non-protective medical intervention, and must be distinguished from knowing a "reality subject to appropriation," as the lawyers say.

If the embryo, or the pre-embryo, is nothing more than a good, morality does not factor (or at least not in the same way) in its utilization, in its destruction, and the law need not deal differently with it than with other goods, including animals. While no one has gone so far as to make this thesis, one can see juridical phenomena with opposing indicators. On the one side: the promotion of the status of animals and the lowering of the status of the *infans conceptus* and of the person in the terminal stage of his existence. On the other side: the personalization of certain (prosthetic) objects and the reification of the person (*infans conceptus*, so-called surrogate mother). Certainly, in many places (for example, France, Canada, the Unites States), doctrinal reflection and sometimes jurisprudence reopen the debate (which was believed to be at this point exclusively concentrated on civil solutions that have to do only with property law) over the juridical status of the conceived baby—prescinding from a consideration of viability, insofar as it is not pertinent and as such is a bogus distinction that establishes among persons various qualitative distinctions that lead logically to eugenics—enlarging the spectrum of this person's rights (the right to therapies, to reparation for damages, to filiation . . .), eventually setting these rights against the other person, for instance, against the mother (the baby's right to care *in utero* against the will of the mother). But there are still various uncertainties, according to which the embryo or the fetus would be simply a potential human person, who nonetheless demands respect. The Instruction of the Congregation reiterates a teaching that relies on the "recent findings of human biological science" on the human character of the fertilized being and, in order to respond to the proposed "becoming," or "potentiality," of this being, it poses a very simple question: "How could a human individual not be a human person?" Lawyers attend: the personality that confers the status of "subject of rights" and not of "object" must be inherent to the character of the individual that begins with the appearance of human life. The ancient "civil death," slavery, actualized a dissociation between individual and person. The juridical examinations to which we have made reference truly have to do with the split between human creature and person. Certain proposed laws in France, in Belgium (along with a proposal for constitutional reform), have also made explicit the reality of the personality of the conceived baby, *in utero* or *in vitro*. The Instruction offers them a true support.

B) The Inadequacy of Self-Regulation

Will these grave issues find a solution in the norms that emerge only from those involved? Such would correspond to the wishes for regulation expressed by certain specialists in medical law, according to whom these issues should have as few legal aspects as possible. But an excessive subjectivism must also be avoided.

1. The Need for Objective Norms

Two traps must be avoided. The first, whose error even the Instruction does not mention, is that of *words*. The expression "pregnancy termination" has greatly contributed to the banalization of abortion; IVF and ET, which might become a proper name as well, will make it easier to accept *in vitro* fertilization and the transfer of embryos. No less dangerous is the substitution of the word "ethical" for that of "moral." Speech about "morality" presupposes that customs must be conformed to higher laws, while speech about "ethics" presupposes that the laws must be conformed to customs. It will perhaps take longer to go from morality *in* situations to a situational morality. Words therefore have a stronger or weaker normative charge.

The second trap is that of the *intention*. Just as sincerity is not truth, so too the intention does not by itself constitute a justifying fact. Criminal lawyers are accustomed to writing that the motivation is generally irrelevant to the occurrence of an infraction, and that principle has been maintained as valid since the last century on matters having to do with medical experimentation. The Instruction, citing *Gaudium et Spes* (n22), confirms that the "moral character of one's behavior does not depend only on the good intention and the evaluation of the motives: the objective criteria must be used." Regarding a particular point, one reads, "But this good intention is not sufficient for making a positive moral evaluation of *in vitro* fertilization between spouses." The intention of the parties involved may be important for bringing it back to the norm (cf. the notion of cause in the request for medical intervention, or even the drawing up of the medical contract); but it is not enough if the object requested, or the means employed, are in themselves illegitimate. Jurists speak in this case of the public order. In reality, the intention that is assumed to be the norm of action and then of judgment practically signifies the abandonment of the norm of law as soon as the mere subjectivity of the individual comes to dictate the law. Now the values we are dealing with here—human life and human dignity—are such as cannot be left to the mere evaluation of those concerned.

Sometimes the excuse for recourse to the sincerity of the intention is found by invoking the *legal vacuum*. In the absence of laws that are applicable to IVF and ET, to surrogate motherhood . . . to what else can we cling? Eminent jurists have already denounced this error—not to say "disinformation." The absence of *specific laws* does not in any way amount to a legal vacuum, if an application can be made to the situations in question from general laws, from the general principles of the law, from the customary solutions, or from jurisprudence. The non-disposability of life and of the status of persons, the repression of voluntary attacks against them, the principle *infans conceptus*, and naturally the principles of a natural law to which certain judgments refer (and to which others, to tell the truth, refuse to apply), and to which the Church certainly refers (the Instruction speaks of "'unwritten laws' etched by the Creator upon the human heart"), vindicate many positions and constitute a juridical framework that is sufficient in itself. To see the law as being merely in specific texts is the result of a positivism whose logical consequence would be to consign human beings into the hands of the legislator. It also entails the vile hiding of a demand, not indeed for a law that is presumed inexistent and the absence of which would generate anguish, but for a new, more permissive, law. Often there are scientists who appeal to this juridical vacuum. Who would have thought that they were so enthusiastic about the law?

2. The Scientist Is Not the Legislator

The President of the Confederation of Catholic Jurists in France, Professor D'Onofrio, said, "Contrary to morality, science is not sufficient to itself; the scientist must go outside his laboratory to investigate his own deontology, since it does not emanate from his chemical solutions, nor can it be derived from algebraic formulas" (November 13, 1985). The Instruction reasserts this idea: "No biologist or doctor can reasonably claim, by virtue of his scientific competence, to be able to decide on people's origin and destiny." And yet the scientist is the one legislating.

First of all, and the theory is a traditional one, eminent biologists and doctors have always reflected on the morality of their professions, they have always recommended deontological behaviors, have denounced perverse procedures. It is important to take these reflections into consideration; they have often contributed to the progress of medical law, which "in its content must express medical morality, at least to the extent of not containing anything opposed to morality" (Pope Pius XII, Speech, September 30, 1954). Secondly, the representatives of the medical profession collaborate with the public officials in order to elaborate the codes of deontology and ensure their application. This is not the promotion of a medical imperialism; the legal profession also retains an objective character; it limits the scientist. However, more recently, since the Declaration of Helsinki in 1964, we see the development of ethics committees, which do not intend to legislate but at the same time are necessarily invested with at least a moral authority, without which their existence could not be understood. Without wishing to pronounce here on the moral worth of their views, which presume an exhaustive and detailed study, it may be asked in what measure these institutions tend to give life to "parallel legislation," whose origins are essentially scientific. The scientific domain promotes its norm of conduct without having received a true and proper delegation for this purpose.

In another sense, one hears biologists lamenting the laws. These appeals are not neutral: they signify on the one hand that the interested parties are by themselves incapable of identifying an objective deontology, and on the other hand that they want the laws tailor-made for themselves, since as soon as that which the law permits is written down, it becomes legitimate. Without explicitly willing it, these scientists are rigorous positivists.

Science is not neutral, states the February 22 Instruction; nor is the law neutral: "Being ordered to man, who initiates and develops them, they draw from the person and his moral values the indication of their purpose and the awareness of their limits." To leave the delineation of norms wholly to the scientists is to risk making morally admissible everything that is technically possible.

Not everything that is allowed is appropriate. "If the legislator responsible for the common good were not watchful, he could be deprived of his prerogatives by researchers claiming to govern humanity in the name of the biological discoveries and the alleged 'improvement' processes which they would draw from those discoveries" (Instruction, III).

This is why public officials, legitimately instituted in view of the pursuit of the common good, must intervene. But within what limits?

II. The Limits of the Intervention by the Public Authority

It might well be asked whether the judiciary authority could be sufficient for the protection of life and human dignity by applying only existing law, or in other words, by inflicting the same penal sanctions that hold for "the law in general." Strangely, although as everyone knows, violations of the rights of the child starting with his conception, contracts contrary to the public order (surrogate motherhood) are being carried out, the judicial processes are case by case, and it is really necessary for an incident to occur (the refusal to return the child on the part of the "surrogate mother") in order for the tribunals to make a pronouncement. It has already been noted that the timidity of the judicial processes in abortive cases constitutes one of the "technical" premises for the preparation for new laws. We return therefore to the work of the legislator.

A) The Purpose of Legislation

"The inalienable rights of the person must be recognized and respected by civil society and the political authority." These rights are, according to the Instruction, that of life and those of the family (cf. the *Charter on the Rights of the Family*, October 22, 1983). "And now We wish to speak to rulers of nations. To you most of all is committed the responsibility of safeguarding the common good. You can contribute so much to the preservation of morals. We beg of you, never allow the morals of your peoples to be undermined. The family is the primary unit in the state; do not tolerate any legislation which would introduce into the family those practices which are opposed to the natural law of God" (*Humanae Vitae*, no. 23).

1. Respect for Life

"The possible recognition by positive law and the political authorities of techniques of artificial transmission of life and the experimentation connected with it would widen the breach already opened by the legalization of abortion."

The protection of life, above all that of the weakest, those most lacking in advocates, with whom even criminals are regularly supplied, constitutes the primary duty of the legislator. Certainly the different juridical systems carry with them the proscriptions for the protection of life, in penal law, in civil law, in medical law; nonetheless, discussions have arisen regarding their applicability to those behaviors that the Instruction takes under consideration.

If the jurists' opinion reveals the inadequacy of this order, the legislator must explicitly prohibit the scientific and commercial use and qualitative selection of embryos and fetuses. Certain legal proposals are geared in this direction. In the same way, the legislator must uphold the prohibition of purely scientific experimentation that is opposed to respect for the principle of totality (cf. Pope John Paul II, Speech, October 23, 1982). One current form of research is that regarding genetic inheritance. Pope Pius XII in his time, Pope John Paul II, and the *Charter on the Rights of the Family* have limited this research to therapeutic purposes, which is what medical law dictates concerning intervention on the person.

2. Respect for the Family

Certain laws abandon, in one way or another, the family institution—as well as parenthood—to individual choice. Different behaviors present the same features and expose the child (whom some dare to call "pre-fabricated") not only to dangers to his future development—dangers that are not well-assessed—but also to the risk of being born with an imprecise parental status. The split between biological parenthood and overt family parenthood, when such becomes a possibility guaranteed by law, threatens the unity and the stability of the family. When third parties become involved—the donors of the gametes, or the womb "provider," or even when one takes the "gifts" of the embryos into account—the baby is no longer the only one to have been considered as an object whom the couple, whether naturally or not, can rightfully claim as they could any public service, but also the third party, whose personality and affectivity are denied and whose body alone matters, is treated no longer as a human but as an instrument. One glimpses the new forms of slavery that may arise as a result. One Canadian magazine published the headline, "Is the Womb a Rentable Space?" As for the baby, it is his right to be conceived and brought into the world in and through marriage, whose unity and solidity have been compromised by manipulative methods of human procreation.

If the international declarations proclaim it an individual's right to form a family and procreate, these rights imply the protection of the legitimate family. The Instruction lays out various exact directives. Were it to depart from these two paths, a piece of legislation would lose its legitimacy, even granting the obligation of tolerating what cannot be prohibited without causing a graver disorder when more important values are not at stake. The more constant teaching limits the legislator's power of intervention. The human being does not belong to him, and therefore, all the more, the person's inherent rights, "by virtue of the creative act from which the person took his origin," do not belong to him either.

B) Resistance to Unjust Law

Redemptor Hominis recalled that the rights of power cannot be founded on anything other than respect for the objective and immutable rights of man, and that law which is contrary to the human good, or even worse, to the divine good, is "unjust." It does not oblige, and, as St. Thomas Aquinas wrote, it becomes more an act of violence than a law. This leads to the problem of resistance to the law, through proportionate means.

1. The Forms of Legal Injustice

First of all, we should examine the evident injustice of the law. Thus, when a legislative proscription authorizes, even only on certain conditions, euthanasia, abortion, non-therapeutic sterilization, recourse to "surrogate mothers," . . . the very wording of the law manifests its contrariness to the fundamental rights of man in his fullness, as the Instruction lays out. To say that those who want to take advantage of these laws can, while those who wish to refrain for reasons of conscience can as well, is a sophism: the legislator is putting objectively illegitimate instruments into the hands of his subjects, which are presented as being on the same level as legitimate means. The neutrality of the legislator is, like that of the scientist, an illusion.

Secondly, there is a more subtle form of legal injustice that is put into practice, which can amount to the preceding. "The civil legislation of many states confers an undue legitimation upon certain practices in the eyes of many today." It is the perversion of the pedagogical value of the law. The fact of a behavior becomes understood, whether in good faith or not, as legitimizing the behavior, which its promoter pretends to tolerate or enclose within certain limits, and it is for this reason that it can be dangerous to legislate in these areas. Even on the best legislative theories, with the best reception of the sense of the law, there remains the recognition of what is in fact a new principle. One understands why the Instruction advises public officials to cultivate an awareness of public opinion. Another subtly unjust law is the one that urges people to commit abortion, etc., for the sake of fiscal or social advantages.

If we consider the situation of the legislator, it is obvious that two forces, otherwise opposed, are likely to pressure him to draft a law contrary to the rights of the child and the family. On the one hand, there are the voices of those who highlight the difficulties of certain particular situations. The law is general; it does not handle very marginal cases by doing something that would lead to a multifaceted effect. On the other hand, there are those who claim that being unable (or unwilling) to establish sanctions means endorsing what happens. Thus one reaches the "conformity of the law with the fact." One could here reference that public authority who complained that ethics has not been updated to match the scientific explosion. At this point, the request for a law becomes merely an excuse; to disobey the law and to do so openly is the work of a visionary legislator!

2. The Forms of Disobedience

It is evident that the Instruction foresees a task in the carrying out of useful reforms, a task that is a doctrinal work, and some authors, including parliamentarians, write on this matter. It is highlighted how, in a traditionally Catholic government, a project for legalizing abortion should have been preventable with the promotion of opposed projects, projects favoring the rights of the conceived baby understood as a human person. The document turns to two other approaches: first of all, the recognition of conscientious objection to such laws.

The Congregation's invitation cannot but be met with approval. All the same, it would be necessary to go beyond the particular settings in which the ability to excuse oneself is recognized, in order to make it a general principle that encompasses all the variable impacts of a law contrary to the rights of man and to the rights of God (laws on divorce, for example; and one knows, with respect to the rejection of divorce, how limited would be the recognition of an attack on religious sentiments when those sentiments are seen to be a result of excessive rigidity). In certain juridical systems, could not the absence of the possibility for conscientious objection be considered as an attack on "fundamental" or "constitutional" rights? We might even see a kind of attack on religious liberty. Following this would be the "passive resistance to the legitimation of practices contrary to human life and dignity." It is not the first time that the Church acknowledges that her subjects, oppressed in their convictions, have the right to resist the law. This doctrine has been affirmed since St. Thomas Aquinas, and the Instruction of March 22, 1986, on *Christian Freedom and Liberation*, while also allowing for the theoretical legitimacy of the final remedy that is armed combat, counseled too this same passive resistance.

This might weaken the force of the laws; but it will strengthen the Law and the value on whose foundation it rests. The various methods may vary according to the legislative systems.

Leaving aside, therefore, the determination of means, with respect to everything else, one finds a constant teaching in the Instruction. Since a law is not a law to the extent that it is not derived from the natural law, and since whatever distances a law from the natural law is a corruption of the law (cf. St. Thomas Aquinas; CDF Declaration of November 18, 1974, on abortion), the struggle against an unjust law is even a duty. "Jurists have this task, than which none is more lofty, of defending within society this universal human worth which is the very source of life, and which is found at the core of not only Christian civilization, of Civilization which is simply and universally human" (Paul VI, Speech, December 9, 1972). The Instruction of February 22, 1987, offers jurists juridical and spiritual weapons of notable significance.

On the Doctrinal Authority of the Instruction *Donum Vitae*

Nearly two years after the publication of the *Instruction on Respect for Human Life in Its Origin and on the Dignity of Procreation* of February 22, 1987, there is a continued increase of interest in the theological debate geared toward a deeper understanding of the document's principles and arguments. The studies, essays, reviews, and commentaries that have been published, both in the Catholic and non-Catholic world, greatly exceed one hundred. In the meantime, biomedical research in the field of assisted procreation progresses at an apparently inexorable rate, improving already existing techniques and proposing new methods, with the intention of overcoming the perplexities and negative effects which have so far been noted.

The Church's intervention, "inspired also by the Love which she owes man, helping him to recognize and respect his rights and duties" (*Donum Vitae*, Introduction, 1), nonetheless continues to find fierce resistance in the widespread technistic and utilitarian mindset, which is unable to comprehend why on earth it should be illegitimate to use a technology that has already managed to produce many hundreds of human beings.

The impact of the cases that have been successful and widely publicized have truly had a dazzling influence, to the point that many remain incapable of accurately perceiving the inhuman logic of a manufactured child. Thus it happens that, even among those who admit that not everything that is technologically possible is automatically acceptable from a moral point of view, there are those who sincerely wonder what is wrong with the effort of achieving a human conception in a manner other than the sexual union of man and woman.

Hesitations and dissents in the Catholic arena have contributed significantly toward complicating matters further. Above all, one cannot underestimate the gravity of the decision by certain Catholic university clinics to continue, on certain conditions, the practice of homologous *in vitro* fertilization. After the clear condemnation present in the document of the Congregation for the Doctrine of the Faith, such a resolution, from the moment in which it was made public, has become a provocation as well.

Those responsible for this very serious rebellion—a rebellion that probably lies outside their intention—continue to justify themselves by claiming to respect the Roman Instruction but not to understand its reasons; they therefore claim not to be in a state to reach that certainty of conscience regarding the illicit character of the use of homologous IVF and ET that they consider a prerequisite for putting an end to the use of such techniques.

Even under these difficult circumstances, there is still the voice of those who have promptly and courageously expressed their clear adherence to the teaching of *Donum Vitae*, making it manifest that the case is all the greater in the case of the public opposition against the Church's Magisterium. Indeed, the issue could not have been interpreted merely as the effort to formulate a personal judgment of conscience in light of a practical determination. The statements of those responsible at various universities, reported by the mass media, even constitute the exposition of a moral doctrine that affirms as legitimate on certain conditions precisely what the Church's Magisterium has declared illegitimate. Such doctrinal dissent is therefore contrary to the right rule of Catholic communion (cf. *Code of Canon Law*, c. 754).

Perhaps it is due precisely to an anticipation of these and other difficulties that in the concluding part of *Donum Vitae* there is included "an invitation with confidence and encouragement to theologians, and above all to moralists, that they study more deeply and make even more accessible to the faithful the contents of the teaching of the Church's Magisterium" (*Donum Vitae*, Conclusion). These words certainly reflect a conscious and realistic preoccupation, not about the logical transparency of the argument presented, and less so about the truth of preceding magisterial teaching, but about the disposition to receive this doctrine in individual and very diverse situations. The concern is well-founded when one considers recent history—which everyone knows—regarding the reception of other documents from the Roman Magisterium on analogous matters, from the Encyclical *Humanae Vitae*—whose twentieth anniversary we mark this year—to the *Pastoral Letter on the Care of Homosexual Persons*, published on the first of October, 1987.

But the aforementioned appeal also reveals a strong awareness on the part of the Magisterium of having reiterated in an explicit, organic, and authoritative way, the doctrinal points—concerning the dignity of the person, the worth of human life, and the nobility of conjugal love—whose teaching appears absolutely essential to the explication of the Church's saving mission. The Church feels, perhaps as never before, a responsibility not only for man's eternal salvation but also for the temporal common good as seen from the perspective of conscience; this common good is actually placed in serious danger both by the escalation of weaponry and by the frenzy of an ever greater dominion over man, which occurs through the control and technological manipulation of the very sources of life. Thus, just as contraception has ended up as an incentive for abortion, it is becoming clear that artificial procreation establishes the operative bases for a cultural preferential option as compared to procreated children (i.e., eugenics).

The *Instruction on Respect for Human Life in Its Origin and on the Dignity of Procreation* could not have been given a more meaningful title. Yet it seems that some people have not recognized it, maybe because they have been so unilaterally struck by the document's severe condemnations with respect to the artificial techniques of procreation, condemnations that have been more hyped by the media. Actually, *Donum Vitae*, by being the current mouthpiece of Catholic doctrine, condemns heterologous artificial fertilization—that is, fertilization using gametes taken from a third party—insofar as it is "contrary to the unity of marriage, to the dignity of the spouses, to the vocation proper to parents, and to the child's right to be conceived and brought into the world in marriage and from marriage" (*Donum Vitae*, II, 2). It also declares surrogate motherhood to be illicit for the same reasons.

As to homologous forms of artificial insemination and fertilization, while recognizing that these are "not marked by all that ethical negativity found in extra-conjugal procreation" (*Donum Vitae*, II, 5), nonetheless, the fact that the conception occurs due to a technical action objectively makes it so that the procreation of the human person—regardless of the intentions of the spouses and doctors—is not the result and the fruit of a conjugal act. It is consequently mutilated in its most natural and specific perfection, since sexual union is the way willed by God for spouses to cooperate with him in the transmission of life to new human persons.

This is why the Instruction declares unhesitatingly that "the Church remains opposed from the moral point of view to homologous *in vitro* fertilization. Such fertilization is in itself illicit and in opposition to the dignity of procreation and of the conjugal union, even when everything is done to avoid the death of the human embryo" (*Donum Vitae*, II, 5).

The Instruction of the Congregation for the Doctrine of the Faith illuminates in a profound and radical way the intimate connection between conjugal love and the generation of children, between human fruitfulness and divine fruitfulness. Human procreation cannot be considered as a kind of physical consequence of love but as something that is part of the dynamic of the spousal gift and that therefore participates in the human person's double dimension, soul and body.

In all truth, such an affirmation—reasserted in the historical moment in which *procreation without sex* has become a reality—cannot be considered an "absolute novelty": it is present in the doctrinal tradition of the Church, and it has been reiterated several times in this century by the pontifical

Magisterium. *Donum Vitae*, in a very timely way, before concluding, counsels, "The precise indications which are offered in the present Instruction therefore are not meant to halt the effort of reflection but rather to give it a renewed impulse," and then immediately adds, "in unrenounceable fidelity to the teaching of the Church" (*Donum Vitae*, Conclusion).

When, failing to observe this principle of sound theological method, one takes a position contrary to a moral doctrine already unequivocally and authoritatively affirmed by the Church's Magisterium, it is either because one fails to recognize the specific competence of the Magisterium *in re morali* or because one fails to accept that such a document has a magisterial character. Now the first option is manifestly erroneous, given what the Magisterium has itself declared quite often regarding its own authority *in moribus* (Vatican II, *Lumen Gentium*, no. 25; Pope Paul VI, *Humanae Vitae*, no. 4; Congregation for the Doctrine of the Faith, *Mysterium Ecclesiae*, June 24, 1973: *Acta Apostolica Sedes* 65 [1973] 401), and it is theologically certain that the Magisterium is competent to make judgments on whether or not a given matter belongs within the sphere of its own competence.

As to the second possibility, the magisterial nature of the *Instruction on Respect for Human Life in Its Origin and on the Dignity of Procreation* may be deduced as much from its form as from its content. Indeed, *Donum Vitae* is a document of a doctrinal nature on moral issues, approved by the pope and legitimately published by the Congregation for the Doctrine of the Faith. As it explicitly states, "During an audience granted to the undersigned Prefect after the plenary session of the Congregation for the Doctrine of the Faith, the Supreme Pontiff, John Paul II, approved this Instruction and ordered it to be published" (*Donum Vitae*).

The Congregation for the Doctrine of the Faith is the first among the Congregations that constitute that organ—the Roman Curia—through which "the Supreme Pontiff usually conducts the affairs of the universal Church . . . which performs its function in his name and by his authority for the good and service of the churches" (*Code of Canon Law*, c. 360). It belongs specifically to it to safeguard the doctrine of faith and morals. And it is "in fulfilling its responsibility to promote and defend the Church's teaching" (*Donum Vitae*, Conclusion) that she has elaborated this document, signed both by the prefect of the Congregation, Cardinal Ratzinger, and by the secretary, Monsignor Bovone.

Even the style of *Donum Vitae* is that corresponding to a document of the authentic Magisterium: it continuously speaks in the name and with the authority of the Church (for example, these significant expressions are used: *The Church's intervention* [Introduction, 1]; *the Church once more puts forward*

[ibid]; *the Church offers* [Introduction, 5]; *the Church . . . forbids* [I, 5]; *the Church remains opposed* [II, 5]; *By defending man . . . the Church of God reminds him* [Conclusion]); and as early as the Foreword, it claims not to "intend to repeat all the Church's teaching on the dignity of human life as it originates and on procreation, but to offer, in the light of the previous teaching of the Magisterium, some specific replies to the main questions being asked in this regard" (*Donum Vitae*, Foreword). In fact, as we have already shown earlier, it demands that previous teaching be upheld, thus consolidating the line of doctrinal continuity and homogeneity.

In this respect, two statements in the Introduction emerge as being particularly indicative: "The Church's Magisterium," says *Donum Vitae*, "does not intervene on the basis of a particular competence in the area of the experimental sciences; but having taken account of the data of research and technology, it intends to put forward, by virtue of its evangelical mission and apostolic duty, the moral teaching corresponding to the dignity of the person and to his or her integral vocation" (Introduction, 1).

And a little later on, the ultimate goal of the document is articulated: "Thus the Church once more puts forward the divine law in order to accomplish the work of truth and liberation" (Introduction, 1), that is, because the promotion of the respect for moral norms is an essential part of her salvific mission.

At this point, therefore, it is impossible to see how one could objectively refuse to give the *Instruction on Respect for Human Life in Its Origin and on the Dignity of Procreation* the obedience of judgment and of practice that the faithful are bound to give the Church's legitimate authority when she presents a doctrine or proscribes erroneous opinions (cf. *Code of Canon Law*, 754).